PRAISE FOR
NEW MOM ESSENTIALS

"I wish Dianna's book had been around when I was going through pregnancy and the first steps into motherhood. She offers an extremely well-researched and thoughtful guide to keeping yourself healthy and sane during this amazing, miraculous and often difficult journey. Highly recommended."

—HEIDI ROIZEN, Partner, Threshold Ventures

"It's overwhelming to be a first-time mom. I remember being inundated with information from multiple sources that I had to sort through on my own. With Dianna's book, moms-to-be will have an integrated go-to resource that is focused on them as a whole person. This guide will empower a generation of happier, healthier, and well-nurtured new parents."

—BETSY ZIEGLER, CEO, 1871

"*New Mom Essentials* underscores the most important part of new parenthood — figuring out what you want for you and your family. Dianna has done the research that parents-to-be and new parents yearn to have at their fingertips. That said, it is her passion to foster a village for expecting parents that most resonates."

—ROB AND DIANA NAGEL, Philadelphia

"I'm impressed that self-care and community care are featured so prominently. We all as a society benefit when we place the care of new parents at the forefront of public health."

—DEMETRIA CLARK, Professional Doula Trainer, Midwife, and Childbirth Educator

New Mom Essentials is like getting pregnancy advice from a wise, knowledgeable, and practical friend. Dianna addresses the most common prenatal and postnatal issues, providing tips from physical and mental health perspectives. In addition to information about diet, exercise, and suggestions for self-care during pregnancy, she shares potential interview questions to ask obstetrician and pediatric providers. This book also offers recommendations for supportive partners looking for ways to help. It is crucial to find and use your voice during pregnancy, and Dianna has tips for addressing family, friends, and even yourself. Terrific, accessible, and clearly-written."

—JACQUELYN MCMILLIAN, PhD, CNM, CNE, Assistant Clinical Professor, Duke University School of Nursing

"A must-give gift for all mothers-in-the-making, who hold our future in their bodies and hearts."

—SALLY BLOUNT, CEO, Catholic Charities of Chicago and former Dean, The Kellogg School of Management

New Mom

ESSENTIALS

A FIELD GUIDE
to BEING YOUR OWN
HEALTH ADVOCATE
THROUGHOUT PREGNANCY
and the FOURTH
TRIMESTER

Dianna He Murray

ISBN: 978-0-578-87845-4 (Paperback)

Library of Congress Control Number: 2021907347

Front cover image © Shutterstock.

Book design by The Book Designers.

Printed in the United States of America.

First printing edition 2021.

Joy & Clarity, LLC

www.joyandclaritylife.com

I dedicate this book to all who take care of moms.

TABLE OF CONTENTS

MEDICAL DISCLAIMER

The information in this resource is not intended or implied to be a substitute for professional medical advice, diagnosis, or treatment. All content, including text, graphics, images, and information contained is for general information purposes only and may not apply to you as an individual. This document makes no representation and assumes no responsibility for the accuracy of information contained, and such information is subject to change without notice. You are encouraged to confirm any information obtained from or through this resource with other sources, and review all information regarding any medical condition or treatment with your physician and other health care providers. Never disregard professional medical advice or delay seeking medical treatment because of something you have read in this resource.

The author does not recommend, endorse, or make any representation about the efficacy, appropriateness, or suitability of any specific tests, products, procedures, treatments, services, opinions, health care providers, or other information in its contents. The author is not responsible or liable for any advice, course of treatment, diagnosis, or any other information, services, or products that you obtain as a result of using this resource.

What is this?
An essentials-based handbook for
pregnancy and the first three months after birth

Who is it for?
New parents-to-be who aren't sure what questions to
start asking and who find all the information online
to be overwhelming *(more on the next page)*

What's the intended benefit?
I hope this resource will uncover some of the
"unknown unknown's" of the pre- and postnatal period,
and that it keeps you focused and stress-free as you
navigate this special season of your life

INTRODUCTION

WHO IS THIS FOR?

This book is for you if . . .

- you want an easily-referenceable handbook, not a novel written in prose

- you're a first-time mom who wants practical information about how to have the best health outcome during your pregnancy, labor, and postpartum

- your partner or someone you love is about to have a baby and you want to know how you can help them to optimize their physical, mental, and emotional health

- you're a physician, doula, midwife, nurse, educator, or other health care provider who cares about supporting the mom in achieving the outcomes she desires

- you want to know what questions to ask, what options to consider, what conversations to have, and how and when to advocate for yourself with regard to the healthcare system and opinionated relatives alike

- you want to take ownership of your health because you know that there aren't enough randomized control trials to definitively know what's best for all women

- you live far away from family and close friends and/or you're worried about how everything will get done after baby arrives

- you recognize that a healthy baby starts with a healthy mother

- you want to take full advantage of your insurance and employer benefits

- you want to see actual examples of what others have done to achieve their optimal health

- you are interested in learning more about a proactive, preemptive approach to health

- you want judgment-free information that will help you make the right choice for *you*

This book is <u>not</u> for you if . . .

- you want a week-by-week guide for what to expect with your body and baby's development during and after pregnancy

- you want information about fertility

- you want to learn how to get your baby to sleep through the night

- you want to know what products to buy or add to your baby registry

- you don't believe in self-care

- you live in a country with parental leave policies, cultural norms, and/or readily-available resources that ensure the mom is taken care of throughout the perinatal period

WHY AM I DOING THIS?

How it started...   *How it's going...*

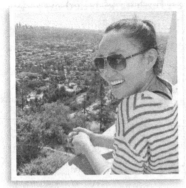 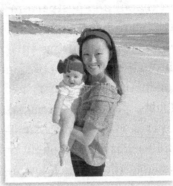

As an immigrant from China, I come from a family of doulas and women's health practitioners. Where I'm from, there is not only cultural support for a postpartum period of "sitting the moon" for Chinese moms, but also a federal-mandated yearlong paid maternity leave. In most parts of the world, there are better parental leave policies than currently exist in the United States. At a time when more women than ever live far away from their closest family and friends, it's no wonder that maternal health outcomes here in America have been declining.

What I believe more than anything else in this world is that without our health, we have nothing. We can't be with the people we love, and we can't do the things we love. As such, I am constantly and continually trying to figure out how to live healthier, and sharing any insights I have with others. Because ultimately, our physical, mental, and emotional well-being dictate not only how we express ourselves, but also how we fulfill our own potential.

So, what does all that have to do with creating this guide? I've spent the last four years of my life trying to answer the question: "What does optimal health look like for women during pregnancy and postpartum?" I even built (and failed at) a digital health startup that aimed to help moms better take care of themselves during this challenging time. After pouring through countless books and research papers, and personally conducting 400+ interviews with doctors, nurses, midwives, doulas, perinatal specialists, therapists, educators, insurance experts, HR benefits managers, new parents, and their family and friends – the thought of just walking away from all of that valuable knowledge I'd gained didn't sit well with me.

A wise friend and mentor once told me that when you're new to something, everything seems simple. As you dive in to learn more, it becomes incredibly complicated. But once you've mastered it, everything can be explained simply again. I am certainly not claiming to be an expert or a master, but my experiences the last few years have left me with the clarity and comfort to be able to take the universe of info I've been exposed to and drill down to what is most essential.

Over the past year, when my friends started sharing the news of their pregnancies and asked me if there was anything from my startup days that might be useful to share with them, I found myself sending them a series of texts, emails, and attachments. So partly for their sake and partly for my own (and now yours, too), I decided to organize it all into what I hope is an easily-digestible resource. My goal is to share the most salient insights from my research so that you can become the best possible advocate for your own health.

WHAT IS A GOOD OUTCOME?

When you ask most people this question, nine times out of ten you'll hear the response, "a healthy mom and a healthy baby." What more could you ask for, right?

But if you're a reader of this book, then chances are, you are not most people. You might be wondering . . . How are "healthy mom" and "healthy baby" defined? By whom? Why are they defined that way? Is there anything I can do to increase my chances of having a good outcome both now and in the future?

Plenty of books exist out there that discuss parenting and pediatric health. And there are many who are much more qualified than I am who have published their theories on what drives poor maternal health outcomes such as postpartum depression and maternal mortality. Even the classification of what is considered a good versus poor health outcome can be hotly contested. One example during labor and delivery is the use of more invasive procedures (e.g., epidural, Pitocin, Cesarean section, episiotomy, assisted extraction) which, if deemed medically necessary, can be lifesaving, but also come with risks that have the potential to pose future health concerns for the mother. What's more is that what is clinically measured (e.g., by healthcare institutions and insurance companies) isn't all that matters. We are whole people, so when I say "health," I mean your whole health, every aspect of it (physical, mental, and emotional), both during this season and for the rest of your life.

The purpose of this book is not to judge how a mom chooses to give birth or what constitutes medical necessity. Rather, it's to give you a heads-up about many of the choices you may not have even known you had. Not only that, but I also want to help you be alert to the kinds of things you can do before baby is born to set yourself up for "health" during pregnancy and long afterward, no matter your circumstances.

KNOW YOUR WHY

"He who has a why to live for can bear almost any how."
—Friedrich Nietzsche

One of the key lessons I've learned from going through this whole journey (both through my research and now as a mom) is that there must be a strong why that sustains your will to see your vision through.

In order to have that optimal health outcome you're hoping for during pregnancy, birth, and postpartum, it helps a great deal to be absolutely clear as to *what* you consider optimal and *why* you consider that to be optimal. There is no "one right way" to give birth. Put aside what "most people" do and think about what it is that *you* want. Once you have clarity around what you want, then it's a matter of figuring out who or what resources and practices can help you achieve your vision.

You might wonder ... "How do I know what I want when I don't know what choices I have?" This book will help illuminate the key decision points and options for you to consider. Once you have your compelling, totally clear, tough as nails *why*, there are many resources (this being one of them) that can help you with the *how*.

HOW TO NAVIGATE AND USE

This book is divided into two sections, each with three parts. For easy reference, each chapter goes into more detail about a stand-alone topic.

1. Prenatal: self-care, crucial conversations, checklist

2. Postnatal: self-care, crucial conversations, checklist

As a field guide, this resource is designed for you to bring to doctor's appointments, to the park, on your morning commute... wherever you are and whenever you find windows of time in your day. No need to read it all in one sitting, and feel free to skip around to what's most salient or interesting. Each topic should only take you a few minutes to read, though the questions, conversations, and thoughts it conjures up may require additional time to work through.

You may notice that the prenatal section has more content than the postnatal section. This is intentional. Make no mistake, the postnatal time often poses many more challenges for moms (new moms, especially). Based on the wisdom shared by many of those I've interviewed over the last few years, this book takes a proactive, preemptive approach to setting you up for success. That means that much of what will help you in postpartum is considered during pregnancy. My hope is that you'll feel so prepared by the time you've finished both sections that you're physically, mentally, and emotionally ready for anything to happen and for anything to come your way. I am woman, hear me roar!

IF YOU TAKE AWAY NOTHING ELSE . . .

The best advice I've been given is to do what's best for *you*.

Throughout this journey, you'll get a lot of people telling you – "you should do this," or "you should do that."

Every pregnancy is different. Every baby is different. Every parent is different.

Take in all the info – both here in this resource and elsewhere – and decide what resonates with you and what doesn't.

Know that whatever you choose to do will be the right thing for you and your baby. You got this!

PRENATAL

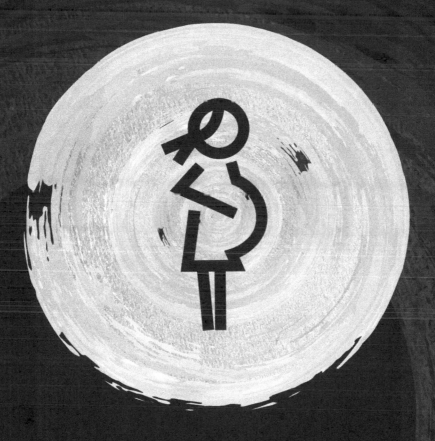

PART I

PRENATAL SELF-CARE

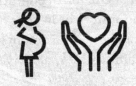

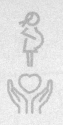

Chapter 1

BUILDING YOUR VILLAGE

We all know it takes a village to raise a child. But in today's world, where most of us don't live next-door to our parents, extended family, and best friends, what's a mother to do?

First, recognize that you can have different people playing different supporting roles in your life:

- Emotional support via phone and video chat from loved ones who live far away

- Social support through new friends you meet in a prenatal yoga or childbirth education class, a new parent's group at work or in your neighborhood, or virtually through Facebook mom's groups and other online communities

- Hands-on support during labor and postpartum from your partner and/or a doula

- Expertise from personal trainers, registered dieticians, lactation/sleep consultants, life coaches, and therapists

- Mentoring from people in your network whose parenting style you admire (e.g., coworkers, acquaintances, friends of friends, members of your church/spiritual center, etc.)

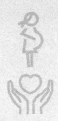

- If you can afford it, hired help in the form of grocery or meal kit deliveries, massage therapists, housekeepers, etc.

Next, accept help when offered. Don't expect to give and take equally. There are different seasons in your life when you may feel like you're receiving more than you're giving – this may be one of them. There will be plenty of opportunities for you to give back later. Consider that it makes others feel good to know they're able to help you – allow them the gift of supporting you in whatever ways they're willing. And if you're still hesitating after reading this, then delegate it – have your partner or another loved one let others know how they can help you when they ask *(or refer them to the next chapter)*.

And finally, be kind to yourself. Treat yourself like you would your best friend if she were pregnant right now. You are enough. You are worthy. If you notice negative thoughts or self-talk creeping in, tell those voices in your head "not today." Instead, turn your mind toward what you're grateful for, or the fact that you are growing a human being inside your belly this very second! How incredible is that?!

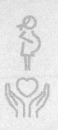

Chapter 2

HOW TO CARE FOR YOUR PREGNANT FRIEND

Most people have great intentions, and when they offer to help, they genuinely mean it. The challenge for many new parents is knowing what to do or what to say when others assume you'll just let them know whenever you need their help. This chapter gives your loved ones concrete ideas for how they can help you most, especially when you either don't know what you need yet or are shy to accept their open-ended offer.

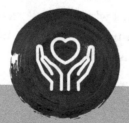

Hi there, friend or family member! I'm reading this book on self-care for moms during pregnancy and postpartum, and thought I would share this page with you since you offered to help. I'm also sharing this with you because, honestly, I don't really know what help I might need, and the author of this book took a stab at describing it for me. Thanks so much for reading and caring!

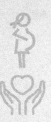

PRENATAL

1. Please resist from repeatedly asking if baby is here. Trust that she will let you know when she is ready. First-time moms, especially, often go past their due date, and she is already dealing with pressure from every direction (including herself) for baby to be here. Your curiosity, albeit well-intentioned, is only going to contribute to her anxiety. If you really can't help yourself and must reach out, just say "thinking of you, and sending love your way!" I repeat. Do NOT keep asking if baby has made a debut.

2. Show her that she matters to you, in your own way. The easiest way is to ask for her baby registry and then get her something she's stated she wants. But that doesn't mean you have to buy a gift if that's not your thing—you could also send a handwritten note, record a funny video, or do something else that speaks from your heart and makes her feel special. Even better? Surprise her with something that's just for her instead of for baby. Ninety-nine percent of people don't do that. You'll definitely stand out, and she'll think it's the sweetest thing ever!

POSTNATAL

3. Be helpful instead of asking how to help. Don't just say, "Let me know how I can help." Most women, even your good friends or family, are not used to reaching out and asking for the help they actually need. Or they may not even know yet how you could help them if they've never before had a kid. Don't put more work on them to figure out how you can help them. Google it. Ask other parents

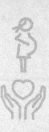

you know for ideas on what you can do and just go ahead and do it. Hint: New moms and partners need food. Lots of it. They also need their laundry done and their house cleaned and their pets walked. They also need to be reminded to practice self-care, so go ahead and offer to babysit so they can take a nap or get their nails done. Although gift cards are a nice gesture, what's even better is if you take it a step further and make the gift an experience. For example, if you want to get her a massage, coordinate with her partner, then book it so that all she needs to do is show up. Be creative. And think about what additional work you would be adding for her with what you say, ask, and do.

4. Be patient with her. Don't forget that this is a sensitive time for new moms. Even more so than during pregnancy, her hormones are all over the place, and she is not the same person you knew before she had the baby. Whatever you might be thinking, withhold that judgment. Try to keep every interaction with her positive. This doesn't mean you should minimize the challenges she may share with you. If you have no idea how to relate, then simply admit that, and tell her "I love you no matter what and you are amazing for bringing this human into the world." Share what you admire about her. Let her know what an incredible mom she is.

5. Be the one to reach out first. Don't expect your relationship to be exactly the same as it was before baby arrived. She still cares about you, but is preoccupied with keeping a tiny human alive at the moment while trying to sneak in as much sleep as possible (which is not much, in case you were wondering.) If you want to see her at all,

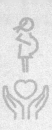

then you may need to make plans around her schedule and come to her neck of the woods to hang out. If you do make plans to meet up somewhere outside her home or via video chat, then don't take it personally if she's late or has to reschedule. She's likely already feeling guilty about it and feeling like she's always apologizing to everyone for not living up to her own expectations for being a good friend or family member. Take that pressure off by proactively telling her it's no big deal, that she's doing great, and that you'll reach back out again in a week or two to see how she's doing. Give her permission to not feel the need to reciprocate or give more of herself (she definitely wants to!) during this season of her life. Right now, it's all about her and her new bundle of joy. Remind her that it's OK to be in a state of receiving, and that there will be another season later on when she can be giving in the way she wants to.

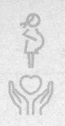

Chapter 3

NURTURING YOUR SPIRIT

On my journey to becoming an executive coach, I had a realization – I had spent a dozen years of my career as a business and strategy consultant for organizations large and small, and yet I wasn't consistently applying that same rigor and clarity of thinking to my own life and career. I've helped many companies and teams articulate their mission, vision, and values, then chart paths toward making them happen. The whole process takes effort, benefits greatly from clear goals, and requires constant prioritization (and re-prioritization). How is this relevant for new moms?

Just as a company starts with defining these things for themselves, we, too, must lay the groundwork to get clear on what we want, how that connects to living our best lives (even while caring for a little one), and create a strategy and plan to close the gap between where we are today and where we want to be. We all hear stories about mom guilt and how hard it can be to stay focused on your path after baby arrives. It's like we can already see it coming – the daily grind of "baby needs this, baby needs that." Will it even be possible to avoid feeling like we're operating from a constant state of whack-a-mole?

Like all hard things, getting clear and staying connected to what *you* want isn't a one-and-done process. It's a lifelong journey

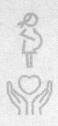

that requires continual inspiration, motivation, and maintenance. Having the big picture in mind of what you're ultimately after will help you keep it all in perspective even though it may at times feel like being a mom is all-consuming. How do you keep from losing yourself in the process?

There is no one-size-fits-all approach. It's best done in partnership with someone you trust – both to bounce ideas off of and to help hold you accountable. However, if you want to dip your toe in the water without doing a deep dive on all that I just mentioned, the following are some reflection questions to get you started.

Make a cup of refreshing fruit-infused water, set aside an hour, and journal what comes to mind. Bookmark this page and revisit these questions as often as necessary until you have clarity.

- What do I want most in life and work?
- What am I most proud of?
- What does success mean to me?
- What do I hope success will mean for my child?
- What am I tolerating?
- What would be different if I truly accepted myself?
- What makes me curious? What gives me energy?
- What motivates me? How do I want to feel?
- Fill in the blank: No one else I know can ___ like I can.
- What am I most grateful for?

"Be you, love you. All ways, always."
—Alexandra Elle

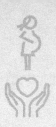

Chapter 4

SAMPLE
RELAXATION TECHNIQUES

As a pre- and postnatal yoga teacher, I'm not only there to help my students practice safe, alignment-based postures, but also to help them stay present and calm the mind. The physical practice of yoga is a moving meditation, but the non-physical aspects of the practice extend far beyond the mat. Below are three of my favorites to guide you in taking a literal "breather," whenever and wherever you might be.

MINDFUL AWARENESS

Close your eyes. Take note of the sounds and ambient noises around you. Now start to notice the soft sound of your own breath, like the sound of ocean waves breaking and receding. Picture yourself sitting on a warm beach, with just the perfect amount of sunshine kissing your forehead and nose, shoulders, arms and fingers, legs and feet. You wiggle your toes in the sand, and look up as you hear the call of a sea bird. You see a few clouds drifting against a clear blue sky. You are enjoying yourself and all that is good in the world. You watch the clouds pass by without attachment. Those clouds are like your thoughts. As thoughts come into your mind, you simply observe, and let

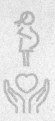

them pass, too, without attachment. You turn your attention back to the sound of the ocean. It smells clean and invigorating. You take another cleansing inhale and exhale.

DIAPHRAGMATIC BREATHING

Sit on an exercise ball or in a comfy chair. Feet are planted firmly on the ground. Rest your hands on your belly. Exhale out fully. Seal your lips gently, and take a deep inhale through your nose. Keep your shoulders relaxed as you visualize your baby getting a big dose of oxygen. On the next exhale, breathe out all of the stressors and "bad air" that don't serve you. Continue for 10 more cycles of breath. Repeat whenever you feel a bit anxious or out of your element.

PROGRESSIVE MUSCLE RELAXATION

Close your eyes. Picture yourself lying on a soft blanket in the middle of a lush forest, one where the sun is casting long beams of light between the trees. You take a scan of your body, and tighten and release each muscle group as you move slowly from head to toe, paying attention to each body part, perhaps spending a little extra time in those areas that need a bit more love or attention. Before moving on to the next muscle group, feel the rush of healing warmth to that part of your body. End by feeling the gravity of the Earth beneath you, supporting and cradling you in its arms as you drift into peaceful slumber.

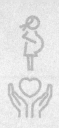

Chapter 5

COMMON
PREGNANCY AILMENTS

What's presented in this chapter are the most common discomforts and relievers I came across in my hundreds of interviews with moms-to-be, obstetricians, midwives, nurses, and physical therapists. Please discuss first with your healthcare provider to determine what may be most appropriate for you in your stage of pregnancy and circumstance.

Nausea/heartburn:
Drink more water between meals, eat bland foods (or what you can stomach), avoid strong smells, eat smaller meals and more slowly, get fresh air, avoid spicy/greasy foods and carbonated drinks, keep head above heart when sleeping

Constipation:
Eat fresh or dried unsweetened prunes and/or drink 100% pure unsweetened prune juice, mix in 1 tsp of flaxseed meal into your smoothie or sprinkle over your meal, consider increasing hydration/movement/fiber intake

Prevent urinary tract infections:
Drink 100% pure unsweetened cranberry juice, ensure good hygiene, consider calling your provider right away for further guidance

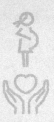

Round ligament pain:
Eliminate jerky movements, bend over or stand slowly and smoothly – planting both feet and evenly distributing weight into your heels, stretch daily (e.g., hamstrings, hips, psoas, quads) and/ or practice prenatal yoga, consider using a support belt

Encourage baby to be head down:
Sit on an exercise ball when seated as much as possible for neutral pelvic alignment, walk daily, do squats and lunges regularly, practice cat/cow

Reduce chance of incontinence and tearing during vaginal birth:
Ask your provider whether or not Kegel exercises and/or perineal massage would be helpful for you

Tone the uterus to encourage more efficient contractions:
Drink 1 cup of 100% organic red raspberry leaf tea daily starting in the third trimester, diffuse clary sage and jasmine organic essential oils starting week 39 to encourage onset of labor (discuss first with your provider and ask about any contraindications)

Encourage cervical ripening and reduce need for medical labor induction/augmentation:
Eat 6 jujubes (unsweetened red dates) daily starting week 36 (discuss first with your provider, especially if you have gestational diabetes)

Carpel tunnel/tingly hands:
Elevate your elbow above your wrist, keep wrists straight and stretch out frequently, avoid repetitive motion, wear a wrist brace (especially at night)

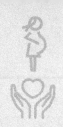

Back pain:
Beware of posture, sit on an exercise ball, practice down dog against the wall, self-massage against the wall with a lacrosse or tennis ball, avoid wearing high heels, avoid standing for extended periods of time, avoid lifting any object over 20 pounds, sleep with a pillow between your legs, consult your provider if you experience back pain that comes and goes (may be contractions or UTI)

Prevent leg cramps:
Mix magnesium oil with lotion of choice and rub into calves, wear compression socks

Treat leg cramps:
Use the padding of your thumb to press firmly into the space between the bow of your upper lips and the bottom of your nose, lift toes up toward shin (dorsiflexion) – helpful if done standing against the wall

Prevent stretch marks:
May be genetic, though rubbing chemical-free lotion on belly starting in second trimester may help (e.g., pure cocoa/shea butter, specially formulated lotions for pregnancy)

Swollen feet:
Soak in warm water with Epsom salt and a few drops of lavender oil, elevate legs and feet

Fatigue:
Get plenty of rest (e.g., take a nap, develop an evening wind-down routine to promote better sleep)

Pregnancy mood swings:
Take a deep breath and ensure that you're getting adequate rest, exercise, liquids, healthy food, and time for yourself and with loved ones

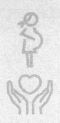

Chapter 6

SAMPLE EXERCISE PRECAUTIONS

The physical activity guidance I consistently heard from the health care practitioners I interviewed is to get into as great shape as you can before becoming pregnant. Being in a healthy BMI (body mass index) range and having a good foundation of moderate exercise (without going overboard) gives you the best chance of staying active throughout your pregnancy, which is good for you and for baby.

PREGNANCY EXERCISE MENTALITY

Gently building up a sweat is good; pushing yourself through pain is not

Aim for getting endorphins and increasing circulation rather than maximizing calorie burn or pushing your body to the limit – just because you can doesn't mean you should

Weight Training: if you weren't doing it regularly before pregnancy, now's <u>not</u> the time to start; for those who did regularly lift prior to pregnancy, now's <u>not</u> the time to go for new personal bests (Note that increased blood volume and extra

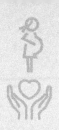

stretchy ligaments due to the hormone relaxin could lead to greater chance of tearing.)

SAMPLE PRECAUTIONS

(The following are based on physically active individuals and low-risk pregnancies.)

Weeks 1-8: no heated yoga or commercial saunas/steam rooms, no contact sports or physical activities with risk of falling (e.g., basketball, bike riding), start or continue 30+ min of cardio daily (e.g., walking, running, swimming, indoor spinning, low impact dance/aerobics, prenatal yoga), no inversions (head below heart)

Week 8+: no direct ab work (planks and other indirect core stability OK), start to practice bending from your hips (instead of your back) to protect your spine, no deep twists or twists that put pressure on your abdomen (to modify, twist only from the rib cage, shoulders, and upper back)

Week 12+: no lying on flat back or on belly (e.g., prop up one hip with pillow while sleeping), no deep forward or backward bends

Week 16+: no weights or heavy objects above 12–20 pounds, confirm with your provider that Kegel exercises are appropriate before starting or continuing (Remember that a healthy pelvic floor involves both muscle tone and elasticity. Strengthening, or contracting, the pelvic floor muscles is important, but learning how to relax and release these muscles is just as important, especially during the pushing stage of birth.)

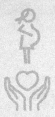

Week 20+: no more planks of any kind

Week 25+: no more running outdoors for those who want to take extra precaution to avoid risk of falling or twisting ankles due to decreased sense of balance as body deals with shifting center of gravity (Note that this is a personal choice, as running is not likely to harm you or your baby, especially if you were a runner before becoming pregnant.)

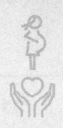

Chapter 7

SAMPLE
NUTRITION PRINCIPLES

There are many schools of thought when it comes to nutrition. While the sample nutrition principles shared in this chapter are evidence-based, have been reviewed by registered dieticians, and have been deemed healthy for pregnancy and beyond by many physicians, please consult a health care professional you trust before making significant changes to your diet.

1. EAT A WHOLE FOOD, PLANT-BASED DIET

Eating a whole food, plant-based diet means you'll naturally get plenty of fiber and be consuming nutrient-dense foods that keep you satiated for a longer period of time. Eat when you're hungry, stop when about 80% full. Prepare ahead of time your healthy snack options so you aren't tempted by the often convenient but nutrient-deficient and empty calories that come from processed and fried food. No raw seafood. No tilefish, swordfish, shark, or king mackerel due to their high mercury levels. If you must eat meat and dairy, choose organic and grass-fed. No lunch meats, pate, smoked seafood, or unpasteurized milk/cheese. Aim to fill at least half of your plate at each meal with vegetables. Soak or wash all produce thoroughly before consuming. Find a good

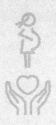

prenatal vitamin and start taking it 3–6 months before conceiving. While you may hear that you're now "eating for two," keep in mind that you're not eating for two adults – just for you and the growing fetus.

2. DRINK LOTS OF WATER DAILY

Drink roughly 8 cups of water every day – more with hotter weather or increased physical exertion. Check the color of your urine – aim for pale or colorless.

3. EAT A VARIETY OF FRUITS AND VEGETABLES IN ALL DIFFERENT COLORS

Eat the rainbow – red, purple/blue, orange/yellow, white/brown, green. These colors occur naturally in produce as a way to let us know they contain disease-fighting nutrients. In general, reds contain lycopene – great for the heart and for reducing cancer risk. Purples/blues contain anthocyanin – great for protecting cells from damage and for reducing cancer, stroke, and heart disease risk. Oranges/yellows contain carotenoids – great for maintaining healthy mucous membranes and eyes. White/brown contain allicin – great for its antiviral and antibacterial properties. Greens contain carotenoids, indoles, and saponins – all of which have anti-cancer properties. There's no such thing as eating too many kinds of dark leafy green vegetables – just make sure they're properly washed, especially if consuming raw. If you meal prep, then know that variety doesn't have to come daily – having the same balanced meals one week, followed by different balanced meals the next week, is just fine.

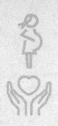

4. LIMIT OR ELIMINATE ALL REFINED SUGAR

Raw fruit is fine. Limit the use of natural sweeteners like stevia, raw honey, blackstrap molasses, 100% pure maple syrup, coconut sugar, and pitted dates. Limit the intake of dark chocolate. Avoid all other sweeteners and processed/packaged foods that contain hidden added sugar.

5. GET A BLOOD TEST

Let your health care provider know that you're planning to conceive, and ask to receive a full physical and blood test. Review the results with your provider to understand where you can improve. Consider making an appointment with a registered dietician to discuss questions and ideas, including any supplements (e.g., prenatal, B12, vitamin D). Remember that our bodies are quite the miracle machine – your body will absorb what it needs from the foods you eat for your growing baby. You just need to ensure that you have nutrients aplenty from which the fetus can draw.

PART II

PRENATAL CRUCIAL CONVERSATIONS

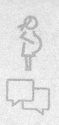

Chapter 8

PREEMPTING MOM GUILT

Setting realistic expectations for yourself and your partner cannot be understated. Your mental health and communication skills will be put to the test after baby arrives, and having conversations in advance about what you will and won't do, what to prioritize or delay will be greatly beneficial when you inevitably start to feel overwhelmed.

If the many moms I spoke to could share some of their wisdom with you, then they would impart, in hindsight, some of the following expectations they wish they had set for themselves:

- "I'm not starving my baby if my milk doesn't come in right away."

- "It's great that others have seemingly neat lives and clean, tidy homes. Comparing leads to despairing. I'm still a good person and a good mom."

- "Taking a shower is not selfish. I don't need to feel guilty for being away from my child to attend to basic hygiene."

- "What I see on social media is only part of someone else's reality. I will focus on what's important for my family."

- "Other people are asking me a lot of questions because they're curious and caring. I don't need to feel pressured

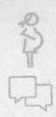

into doing things a certain way. I don't need to have figured out when I'm going back to work, how long I plan to breastfeed, or when and if I plan on having another child. It's ok to not have all the answers. We will figure it out as we go."

- "It's completely normal for me to be very hormonal after birth. I am the best mother for my child. We will learn and grow together as a family."

- "My baby will not be predictable no matter how many manuals I read on infant sleep, milestones, etc. I can take each day as it comes and will become a better parent because of it."

- "At times, it might feel like everything is falling apart. Our house is messy for several months at a time, the laundry is left for too long in the washer and needs to be rerun, the dishes are still in the sink, there are a dozen fixtures and appliances in need of repair, and everything feels like it's in disarray. We will get around to all of it eventually, even if we don't know when that might be. Life will not be the same in ways we can't yet fathom, and we're setting ourselves up for failure if we expect to keep all these plates spinning."

- "I am _not_ doing everything wrong. This is new. Like anything new, there is a learning curve. I am adaptable and resilient, and I am a wonderful mother."

- "People may or may not tell me that I'm doing a good job or give me any indication that they recognize how much I do for my child. _I_ know, and my child benefits tremendously from my love. That's all that really matters."

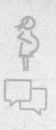
Why is this part of the "crucial conversations" section of this book, you might ask? Because this is one of the most important conversations you can have with yourself. Our inner talk tracks can be more critical than anything we would ever say to anyone else. We owe it to ourselves for that inner voice to be kind.

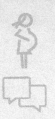

Chapter 9

HOUSEHOLD PLANNING

We've all heard the adage that failing to plan is planning to fail. This is especially true when it comes to division of labor pre- and post-pregnancy. Some questions you may want to consider in creating the household plan include:

- Who does what now? How often? (e.g., grocery shopping and meal prep, financial management, cleaning, laundry, trash/recycling, car/yard maintenance, plants/ pet care, etc.)

- What changes after baby arrives? Who does what then? How often?

- What are our plans for parental leave? Who needs to go back to work first?

- Will we have support (e.g., family and friends, hired help)? What's our back-up plan?

- Who has primary responsibility for each task/chore?

- How often do we plan to check-in on (and potentially revise) the task/chore list?

The following are a few ideas for how well-intentioned loved ones can help when they ask:

- Share your list of household to-do's and let them volunteer to take over anything they like

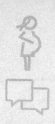

- Suggest a time (recurring or not) for them to come over to take the baby out for a walk in the stroller (Bonus: Pick a window between feedings so mom can get a nap in!)

- Let them know that food is always welcome and very much appreciated!

Below are tips from other parents when planning for visitors and communicating pregnancy news/progress:

- It might be hard to know in advance how you'll feel about visitors, but know that you don't need to feel guilty for setting boundaries. Anticipating potential challenges with certain family members and discussing in advance how to address them will help everyone involved. It may even be worth designating a point person for all visitor management considerations once baby arrives.

- One way to avoid the barrage of questions is to delay sharing the news about your pregnancy. With more people working remotely, it's become a bit of a trend to wait until the six-month mark to spill the beans. Consider telling friends and coworkers that your due date is two weeks later than it is – no need for extra pressure (even if unintended) from well-meaning acquaintances constantly asking when baby will arrive.

- Consider also keeping it from extended family when you're in labor or on the way to the hospital/birth center. Or, at least, if you do let them know, be prepared for the grandparents-to-be (especially if this is their first grandchild) to constantly text and/or call for progress updates. It's only natural – they'll very likely be worried and anxious and excited and anything but patient. Can you blame them?!

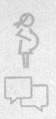

Chapter 10

NAVIGATING RETURN TO WORK (OR NOT)

OK, let's be honest. Our parental leave policies here in the U.S. really suck. Given that reality, what can we do about it, especially if we actually enjoy our job or don't have the financial means to leave?

For large employers, your ability to negotiate a policy exception with HR may be limited. But that doesn't mean you should throw in the towel and think your options are either to be torn away from your baby right away or to quit.

Or, you may find yourself in a situation (like a few of my friends did) where you work for a smaller employer with no parental leave policy – leaving you with the onerous task of having to research and draft it yourself, then convince leadership to adopt your proposal.

Alternatively, you may find yourself in the fortunate position where you have the means to leave your job, but find yourself asking: "What's the impact of leaving on my overall career or lifetime earning potential? How long can I take time off from work and still be competitive and employable? What's best for me *and* my family? What do I think will be most fulfilling now *and* later?"

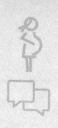

You're probably not surprised to hear that there's no one-size-fits-all solution. How we each deal with these (and other unique personal circumstances) will vary widely. However, it does help to figure out the following . . .

1. What is your ideal postnatal work scenario? Be specific.

- *For example, if you want to stay*: Do you want to come back to the office right away or work remotely for a period of time? Do you want to come back full-time or switch to part-time, then ramp-up responsibilities as you feel ready?

- *For example, if you want to leave*: Do you want to be a stay-at-home parent, find remote or part-time work in another field, start your own business, or ultimately return to your previous career full-time? How will you know it's time to do something different, if that's your desire? What do you require to feel comfortable (even happy) with your decision?

2. What's the best way to communicate your ideal scenario with others in a way that maximizes your chances of getting what you want?

- *For example, if you want to stay*: What's in it for your boss and/or team? Consider their perspectives, and creatively think about ways you could work with them (and possibly others) to develop a win-win solution.

- *For example, if you want to leave*: What do you need to do now, if anything, to set yourself up for future success in your chosen path or endeavor?

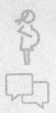

3. Who or what could help as you navigate these choices?

- Whether you're leaning one way or another, it can be helpful to talk to other parents about the choices they've made. Here are a few questions you could consider asking:

  - What were you optimizing for when you made your decision?

  - What creative arrangements did you come across as you were making your decision?

  - If you could go back and have a redo, what would you do differently?

- **Additional Resources:** *Crucial Conversations: Tools for Talking When Stakes Are High* (Patterson et al), *Getting to Yes: Negotiating Agreement Without Giving In* (Fisher et al), *Bargaining for Advantage: Negotiation Strategies for Reasonable People* (G. Richard Shell), *Negotiate Without Fear: Strategies and Tools to Maximize Your Outcomes* (Victoria Medvec)

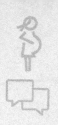

Chapter 11

RELEASING YOUR FEARS

In the 1920s, British obstetrician Dr. Grantly Dick-Read described what has become known as the "Fear-Tension-Pain" cycle. He suggested that fear causes a woman to become tense (e.g., increased adrenaline, ineffective contractions), and that tension increases pain (e.g., decreased oxytocin, endorphins, and blood flow to the uterus). The increased pain, in turn, increases fear (e.g., decreased pain threshold), and the cycle repeats.

In order to release our fears, we have to first name them and identify their source. The following exercise may help.

FEAR RELEASE EXERCISE

1. Set aside 30–60 min with your partner (or a loved one) and individually write down your answers to the following:

    a. What was my own birth like? What impact does this and other birth stories I've heard have on my thoughts about our baby's birth? What expectations do I have? What assumptions am I making as a result?

    b. What is my idea of the kind of support I'll need throughout pregnancy and after baby arrives? How could I get the support I need?

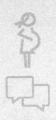

c. Is my marriage/relationship secure, loving, and mutually nurturing? What needs do I have or anticipate having?

d. Will I be able to continue to pursue my own goals? What will need to change, if anything? Does my partner support me in my goals to return to work or stay home with the baby? How do I anticipate this will affect our relationship?

e. Is there space in our home for baby? What accommodations will need to be made?

f. What's my level of comfort, confidence, and trust with my provider(s)/care team? Do I feel they are supportive of my birth plan? Have I made my wishes known?

g. Am I concerned at all about finances being stretched as a result of adding another person to our family?

h. How do I feel about the effect that baby will have on my life (e.g., excited, overjoyed, anxious, concerned)? What's making me feel this way?

i. How do I typically deal with uncertainty or ambiguity? What do I think will help me let go of the need to know and/or control any given situation during pregnancy and after baby is here?

j. What, if any, traumatic memories or experiences are still affecting me?

k. What unspoken expectations do I have for myself, my partner and/or others? What assumptions have I made about what others expect? (e.g., during pregnancy, about how I will give birth, regarding sexual intimacy, from me as a parent)

l. What is causing the most concern or anxiety for me right now?

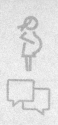

m. What will be most effective in releasing my fears and anxiety? Who or what could help me along the way?

2. Once complete, take turns sharing your answers to each question.

3. Debrief for 15–30 min on what you learned about yourself and each other, as well as how you can best support each other going forward. Discuss what, if any, professional help and resources may be needed.

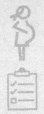

- Take a **childbirth education class** (either online or in person) to start mentally preparing for labor and delivery

- Create **birth plan** and share with prenatal care team (including discussing in detail how your partner and/or a doula can support you during birth and parental leave; note that some doula services may be covered by your insurance)

- Start thinking about **childcare options**

- **Interview and select pediatrician(s)**; add provider contacts to phone

- **Install car seat** (or call your local police/fire department to inquire if they can help or inspect to ensure proper installation based on the latest safety standards; note that this should always be free of charge)

- **Become familiar with essential baby items** before delivery day (e.g., open packages, read through instruction manuals, buy batteries/charge items, download apps)

- **Pack a bag for delivery day** (or gather items for ease of use if choosing a home birth)

- **Assemble key passwords and info** you'll need for after baby arrives (e.g., device and account logins for baby apps, phone numbers, emergency contacts, etc.)

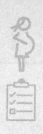

Chapter 13

INSURANCE
AND HR BENEFITS

Call your insurance company sometime in your first trimester and tell them you're pregnant. Then, ask them what info they tend to share with those who are pregnant, as well as what they need from you when. (e.g., prior authorizations for genetics or gestational diabetes testing and/or post-delivery hospital stay, protocol for adding baby to your insurance, any coordination of benefits requirements you should know about so that you're not blindsided by things like the birthday rule)

WHAT IS THE BIRTHDAY RULE?

Depending on which state you live in, most insurance companies will have this in place to determine who pays the bills and in what order if a child has double health insurance eligibility. It's called the birthday rule because whose policy pays is based on which parent's birth month and day comes first in the calendar year.

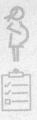

Be sure to ask what resources are available to support you in pregnancy and postpartum. You may qualify for some of the following:

- Durable medical equipment (e.g., hospital-grade, electric and manual breast pumps and replacement parts; home blood pressure monitor; pulse oximeter, body weight scale, and/or activity tracker) – note that some or all of these may require a prescription

- Access to professional expertise (e.g., nurse concierge or hotline; doula, social worker, mental health, and/or coaching support; nutrition, breastfeeding, and/or childbirth education; lactation and sleep consultant services)

- Access to third-party pre- and postnatal support and telehealth services (e.g., Maven, Ovia)

- Note: Some individuals and families may qualify for additional government assistance. Contact your insurance company to learn more about the availability of community programs and help with food, housing, and economic insecurity, transportation, and other resources. (e.g., Special Supplemental Nutrition Program for Women, Infants, and Children (WIC), www.fns.usda.gov/wic)

Depending on the nature of the relationship between your insurance company and your employer, you may have to **call your employer's HR benefits center** separately to ask about some of the above in addition to the following:

- Policies regarding time off (including parental leave, short-term disability, FMLA, sick leave, vacations and holidays)

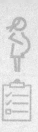

- Policies regarding remote work or changes in job status (e.g., switching to part-time work, paid or unpaid sabbaticals)

- Support for breastfeeding after returning to work (e.g., refrigeration and storage, mother's rooms for pumping, shipping services such as Milk Stork)

- Other perks, discounts, and gifts for employees (e.g., fertility benefits, gift cards for food delivery services, on site or sponsored daycare, product promos or rentals such as the SNOO Smart Sleeper baby bassinet, reduced fees for childbirth education, reimbursement for fitness equipment and/or classes, etc.)

WHAT IS THE DCFSA?

DCFSA stands for Dependent Care Flexible Spending Account. It allows you to set aside money tax-free to pay for eligible dependent care services (e.g., daycare, in-home care). Now this is *really* thinking ahead, but if you have the option, then it's worth doing the calculation during your annual benefits open enrollment period to see if you would benefit by using the DCFSA to reduce your taxable earnings.

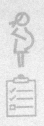

Chapter 14

SAMPLE
PARENTAL LEAVE (U.S.A.)

As of the writing of this book, there is no federal-mandated paid parental leave in the U.S., and only a few states mandate any paid parental leave at all. The Family and Medical Leave Act of 1993 (FMLA) requires twelve weeks of unpaid leave annually for mothers of newborn or newly adopted children if they work for a company with 50 or more employees. In 2019, the Federal Employee Paid Leave Act (FEPLA) was put into place, which grants federal employees up to twelve weeks of paid leave for the birth, adoption, or fostering of a child. What about everyone else? The answer remains to be seen for now. For non-government workers in America, the bottom line is that paid leave (or even unpaid leave with your job guaranteed) is largely up to your employer to decide.

Below is what parental leave looked like for me and my husband in the state of Illinois in 2020 . . .

FOR MOM

(Maximum leave allowed = 14.5 weeks)

1. Paid time off (PTO)   Mandatory 1 week PTO during short-term disability waiting period

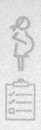

2. Short-term disability (STD)	5 weeks paid at 60% of base salary, to be used immediately upon delivery (else forfeited altogether)
3. Paid parental leave	6 weeks, must be used consecutively within 6 months of delivery
4. Unpaid FMLA	None, since FMLA runs concurrently with STD and parental leave (Check the latest laws for family medical leave in your state.)
5. Paid time off (PTO)	Remaining 2.5 weeks PTO, to be used only with HR and manager approval since FMLA has been exhausted

FOR PARTNER

(Maximum leave allowed = 12 weeks)

1. Paid parental leave	2 weeks
2. Paid time off (PTO)	No limit, but not encouraged
3. Unpaid FMLA	10 weeks, but not encouraged (This is a maximum of 12 weeks, inclusive of all other time off.)

If you're lucky, here's what your employer may allow:

- 6-12 months paid parental leave or sabbatical
- Flexible return-to-work arrangements (including remote work and/or part-time ramp up options)

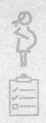

Chapter 15

ASSEMBLING
YOUR CARE TEAM

Once you have an idea of how you'd like to give birth and have toured a few local facilities, it's time to assemble your prenatal care team. This may or may not include a physician or midwifery group, labor/postpartum doulas, and/or independent providers who can be consulted ad hoc for a second opinion.

- It's worth taking a look at the questions below prior to contacting providers and **doing some research to develop a sense of your own birth preferences and beliefs**. Don't be afraid to interview multiple providers. How they react to being questioned (not just their responses) reveals a lot about how they'll be with you should you choose them. (If you feel bullied or talked down to now, then chances are that will only continue!)

- If breastfeeding is important to you (and you plan to give birth outside your home), then it may be worth finding a birth center or hospital designated as "baby friendly." (For more information, see www.babyfriendlyusa.org.)

Below are some questions to consider asking a prospective health care provider for pregnancy and labor/delivery:

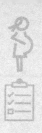

1. **General Philosophy**: What are your core values, priorities, and goals? How do you feel about your birth preferences and/or birth plan? How would *"a particular health condition/concern"* affect the care you provide and recommend? (See the *Creating Your Birth Plan* chapter for additional considerations.)

2. **Logistics**: What is your education/certification? How long have you been practicing? How many births have you attended as the primary attendant? Do you practice alone or with others? (What are other team members' experiences and backgrounds? Do they share your philosophy of care?) When are your planned vacations in the next 12 months? What are your office hours? How often would I see you for appointments during pregnancy and postpartum?

3. **Routine Practices**: What are your protocols for care during pregnancy and during each stage of labor and delivery? How do you define and handle complications? How do you monitor the well-being of the baby during labor? (e.g., continuous electronic fetal monitoring, handheld doppler, fetoscope/stethoscope) What are the pros and cons of the way you choose to monitor the baby? What positions do you recommend for birth? What is your usual approach if labor is progressing slowly? How would you recommend that I prepare for managing pain during labor and birth? What other pain medications are options? What drug-free measures for pain relief are available where you practice? Do you support vaginal delivery for breech babies, multiples, or vaginal birth after cesarean (VBAC)? What happens if baby is past due or breech? How do you feel about doulas, labor assistants, or family and friends being present during labor and delivery? Is video or still photography allowed? What is your approach to newborn care? What

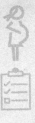

are the routine procedures for a healthy baby? What kind of postpartum care and/or support can I expect?

4. **Interventions**: Under what circumstances do you recommend induction, IVs, continuous fetal monitoring, Pitocin, episiotomy, forceps or vacuum, C-section, or immediate clamping of the umbilical cord? What is your rate of each of these within your practice? How does that compare to the rate at the hospital/birth center where I'll deliver?

    - <u>If important to you</u>: How many unmedicated/natural births have you attended? Do you support my ability to be active and move around during labor – why or why not? Do you support my choice to eat and drink during labor? How do you feel about a water birth? What is your view on elective inductions and/or scheduled C-sections? What mother-centered options do you offer for C-sections? (e.g., maternal assisted C-section, no screen to obstruct view, delayed/no cord clamping, immediate skin-to-skin contact after birth, breastfeeding in recovery) What support can I expect to receive for breastfeeding?

    - <u>For home births or birth centers</u>: Are you licensed and certified? What do you require to accept patients to give birth at home? Do you have a formal agreement with an obstetrician to provide care if complications occur? What is considered an emergency, and what do you do if one were to arise? Under what conditions would I be transferred to a hospital? What is your hospital transfer rate? Which hospital(s) would I be transferred to and is it covered under my insurance plan?

5. **What makes your practice unique compared to others?**

6. **What other questions should I be asking?**

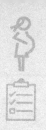

Chapter 16

STANDING
UP FOR YOURSELF

Hopefully this goes without saying, but being pregnant and giving birth are natural things your body is born knowing how to do. You are not sick. There is not something wrong with you. And you are most certainly not a patient with a disease.

In an ideal scenario, your care team fully supports your vision while bringing to light important evidence-based practices as your health care experts and partners. Even so, it's important that we realize we have ownership of the decisions made throughout. It's one thing to want to turn over all responsibility for decision-making to the experts (which many people do and are fine with). But it's another thing altogether to feel pressured into decisions that affect you and/or your baby differently than what you had imagined and be powerless in standing up for what you want.

If you are one of those people who would rather know what you're getting into and why, then it's crucial to ask questions and research your hospital/birth center's policies throughout your journey to parenthood. Know that it's not just "follow the policy or you're out." It may even be the case that some providers don't personally agree with certain standard policies,

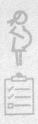

but unless you explicitly ask how it could be done differently in your situation, they won't share any alternative options with you other than "the norm."

Later on, we'll get into specific questions you can ask using the B.R.A.I.N. framework to vet decisions. But essentially with every decision, you want to weigh the benefits, risks, alternatives, your instincts, and what-ifs should you decide to take no action or delay action. Remember that very rarely will it be the case that you have absolutely no choice and no say in the matter.

Medicine is both an art and a science. The science is evidence-based research that provides best practices for what to do the majority of the time. The art is how your care team individualizes that body of research for you. It's important for patients and their providers to develop trusting relationships, and in the case of pregnancy, childbirth, and postpartum care, developing that degree of trust is vital. Of course, it takes effort by both sides to foster trust, and the earlier you're able to discuss with your providers your options, the better. *(See the Creating Your Birth Plan chapter for a sample list of options to explore.)* That way, you can get a sense for whether or not your conversations are moving forward in a way in which you feel comfortable. Feeling free to ask questions is a fair expectation to have, and the right providers for you will partner with you so that you feel heard and supported.

Even if you've assembled a team of providers you feel confident in and trust, it may still be the case that you go into labor at a different facility with a different care team than originally planned (due to travel or other reasons outside your control). Whether it be related to pregnancy, labor and delivery, postnatal recovery, or breastfeeding – in situations in which there are

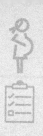

staff who are unfamiliar with you and have different philoso-phies of care with regard to you or your baby, the following may help you get on the same page . . .

- "I'm wondering – can you help me understand what other options there are?"

- "Can you please explain the risks of doing what you're suggesting?"

- "Thank you for your advice, but we need some time to think about it."

- "I'd like to call my provider. Can you please repeat what you just said to them?"

- "I have just spoken with my provider, and am fully aware of the benefits and risks. I am choosing to do ___ at this time."

- "I'm feeling very uncomfortable with this. How would you suggest we reach a joint decision here?"

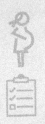

Chapter 17

SAMPLE PRENATAL APPOINTMENT SCHEDULE

How much you should expect to pay for labor and delivery varies widely based on your employer, your selected insurance plan and its negotiated rates with in- and out-of-network providers, whether or not you qualify for government assistance, how and where you choose to deliver, and, of course, your personal birth circumstances. Your employer may offer benefits counseling (e.g., ALEX by Jellyvision), but in case you're curious what you (and your insurance dollars) are paying for, here is a visit-by-visit breakdown of what routine care looks like for a low-risk pregnancy with a midwifery group at a Chicago-area hospital in 2020. All care was in-network under a health savings account (HSA), preferred provider organization (PPO) plan.

	WEEK	ROUTINE CARE	OUT-OF-POCKET COST
TRIMESTER 1	**WEEK 6**	· Urine test to confirm pregnancy · Interview providers and select care team	$77 for urine test

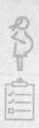

	WEEK	ROUTINE CARE	OUT-OF-POCKET COST
TRIMESTER 1	**WEEK 8**	· Nurse education visit: intro to the practice, family and medical/immunization history, initial gauge of birth preferences, description of optional tests during pregnancy and required insurance prior authorizations · 9 tubes of blood drawn to establish a baseline for everything	$800 for blood work and labs
	WEEK 12	· First prenatal visit: urine sample, weight, blood pressure, handheld doppler · Annual physical and gynecological exam, pap smear · Guidance to supplement with vitamin D based on lab results	$142 for initial health care provider consultation

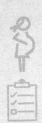

WEEK	ROUTINE CARE	OUT-OF-POCKET COST
WEEK 16	· Urine sample, weight, blood pressure, hand-held doppler · Optional childbirth class registration · Reminder to register for baby's birth (required by local hospital)	
WEEK 20	· Anatomy ultrasound · Prenatal appointment cancelled due to COVID-19 (would have been: urine sample, weight, blood pressure, handheld doppler, fundal height)	$532 for anatomy ultrasound
WEEK 24	· Urine sample, weight, blood pressure, hand-held doppler, fundal height	

TRIMESTER 2

	WEEK	ROUTINE CARE	OUT-OF-POCKET COST
TRIMESTER 3	**WEEK 28**	· Gestational diabetes test (1 hr fast) · Complete blood count (CBC) · Urine sample, weight, blood pressure, hand-held doppler, fundal height · Guidance for tetanus/ diphtheria/pertussis (TDAP) vaccination (option to decline)	$60 for blood work and labs
	WEEK 30	· Urine sample, weight, blood pressure, hand-held doppler, fundal height · Reminder by provider to start looking for pediatrician	
	WEEK 32	· Video visit due to COVID-19 (would have been: urine sample, weight, blood pressure, handheld doppler, fundal height)	

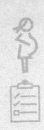

	WEEK	ROUTINE CARE	OUT-OF-POCKET COST
TRIMESTER 3	**WEEK 34**	· Video visit due to COVID-19 (would have been: urine sample, weight, blood pressure, handheld doppler, fundal height)	$0 for electric and manual breast pumps, $0 for hospital grade breast pump rental with prescription (all fully covered by insurance)
	WEEK 36	· Growth ultrasound · Urine sample, weight, blood pressure, handheld doppler, fundal height · Group B strep (GBS) culture	$66 for GBS test, $1,098 for growth ultrasound
	WEEK 37	· Urine sample, weight, blood pressure, handheld doppler, fundal height	
	WEEK 38	· Urine sample, weight, blood pressure, handheld doppler, fundal height · Option for complete blood count (CBC) done in advance to avoid blood draw on delivery day	$12 for CBC

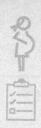

	WEEK	ROUTINE CARE	OUT-OF-POCKET COST
TRIMESTER 3	**WEEK 39**	· Urine sample, weight, blood pressure, hand-held doppler, fundal height · Option to check cervical dilation	
	WEEK 40	· Non-stress test · Urine sample, weight, blood pressure, hand-held doppler, fundal height · Option to check cervical dilation · Option for manual cervical stimulation	$105 for non-stress test
	WEEK 41	· Non-stress test · Ultrasound to check amniotic fluid · Urine sample, weight, blood pressure, hand-held doppler, fundal height · Option to check cervical dilation · Option for manual cervical stimulation	$84 for non-stress test, $0 for hospital birth and 2-night stay after reaching out-of-pocket maximum (insurance paid $8,425 for vaginal delivery)

The information in this chapter is meant to be illustrative only, and may not be used as a reliable source for healthcare pricing, which varies based on many factors. Depending on your personal situation and circumstances, your provider(s) may choose to administer a very different plan of care than the example provided here.

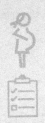

Chapter 18

IS NATURAL
BIRTH FOR YOU?

What does natural birth even mean? Don't Google it, please. Or do, and be prepared to be super confused. For some, the term "natural" simply connotes a vaginal delivery. For others, it means that there was no medical intervention used in labor and delivery. Certainly, associating a "normal" birth with a "natural" birth can feel like an affront to a mom who wanted one but couldn't and downright patronizing to a mom who was perfectly happy with a planned Cesarean.

Many health care practitioners shy away from using the terms "natural" and "normal" altogether. Instead, those who are woman-centered will want to support the mom-to-be in achieving the birth she desires while practicing evidence-based medicine. However, there is often an underlying assumption that the mom knows what kind of birth she desires. Where does a first-time mom even begin?

You might have heard horror stories or grown up with a certain image of childbirth, and may be absolutely terrified of the pain you're about to experience. Hollywood has a way of capturing and selling drama well. You may have also heard that there are women out there who were able to give birth without the use

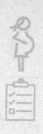

of medication or clinical intervention. That must be an urban myth, you say to yourself. You know you're not going to get a trophy for turning down the epidural, yet you also wonder . . . Why is it that some moms still choose to have an unmedicated birth? Is that even possible for someone like me?

Those are good questions. In short, the thought behind preparing for a birth with minimal medical interventions is both to increase the probability of an easier postnatal recovery and to reap the full benefits of natural hormones released during the process to aid with baby bonding and starting to breastfeed. It might not surprise you to learn that it costs less, too (often on the scale of 50–100%+ less).

Let's look at a scenario I've heard one too many times. A mom-to-be is induced for labor. She feels that the contractions are unbearably strong, and decides to get an epidural for the pain. Labor takes a long time, especially for first-time moms. Something unexpected happens (e.g., failure to progress, fever, baby is in distress, etc.), and the mom ends up having a vacuum extraction, forceps-assisted delivery, or emergency C-section. How likely is it that this scenario will happen to you? That not only depends on your particular situation, but also on the historical intervention rates of your care team, the hospital or birthing center and its labor and delivery policies.

It's not the end of the world if these things happen. Clinically-speaking, chances are that mom and baby would still be considered physically healthy if an intervention was used. But what happened, and could the cascade of interventions described here have been avoided? The circumstances very much depend on each woman's individual situation. What this example does highlight, though, is the need to consider what risks you're

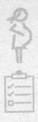

willing to take and why. This is why some low-risk moms choose to turn down induction or painkillers, because they know that the female body is physically capable of birthing a child and they don't want to introduce any outside elements that might mess with that. In other words, they know the odds of the above scenario happening to them based on their choice of provider and location, and have decided that they would like to minimize those odds.

Given all this, you might be wondering, "If it's a win for the health of mom and baby and a win for lowering overall health care costs, then why don't more women attempt an intervention-free birth?" The two most common reasons are because their provider (or other voice of authority that they trust) doesn't present this as a viable option or questions why they're even considering it. With certain high-risk pregnancies and other complications, it may be that trying for an unmedicated birth just isn't advisable. But don't let that be conflated with a provider's dismissal of your questions about the short- and long-term implications of the available options and/or his or her proposed path of care.

While women have had to give birth without medical intervention for hundreds of thousands of years, modern medicine has come up with pretty good ways of making the whole process a bit more comfortable. We now have the ability to save the life of a mother and child via surgery and other procedures, for example. When medically necessary, it's really quite remarkable what technology can now do to help. But no amount of medicine or technology can replicate your body's innate ability to produce a human being – at least, not yet. An unmedicated birth may not be possible (or even desirable) for all women. On the flip side, no one can argue that for many women, an unmedicated birth is perfectly safe and appropriate.

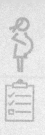

As part of ensuring you are equipped to be your own best health advocate with regard to the birthing process, I want you to walk away empowered with the knowledge that it is absolutely within your rights to ask any health care professional for clarification and justification until you understand the full implications of the recommendations. No one is able to escape some sort of bias, medical practitioners included, and the more confident you are in asking the questions that help align your desires with your provider's philosophy of care, the more you increase the odds of an optimal outcome for you and your growing family. Childbirth requires physical, mental, and emotional preparation, no matter how you end up giving birth. Doing the legwork now during pregnancy (or even beforehand if you're so inclined) allows you to have eyes wide open whether or not you choose to pursue your definition of a "natural" birth. And with that, onto birth planning!

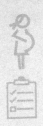

Chapter 19

CREATING
YOUR BIRTH PLAN

Mom's Name:
Mom's Date of Birth (DOB):
Baby's Due Date:
Insurance Info:
Birth Partner's Name (e.g., husband, doula):

Family Physician's or
Pediatrician's Name and Contact:

BIRTH PREFERENCES
    I would like the following:

    Please discuss with me first before
    any of the following:

While we may generally associate labor and delivery with being a very physical endeavor, it is actually very much a mental and emotional one as well. In creating a birth plan, there are two primary things to keep in mind. First, do the research to know what your preferences are and what would make you feel most comfortable. And second, be flexible. By having open discussions with trusted providers well before birth day happens, you'll better be able to navigate changes as a team should you need to adjust your plan.

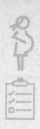

Below are potential decision points to consider. Remember to use B.R.A.I.N. when thinking through your options.

> **The B.R.A.I.N. Framework for Decision-Making:**
>
> B = Benefits; What are the benefits?
> R = Risks; What are the risks?
> A = Alternatives (or other options); What alternatives
>   are available?
> I = Intuition/Instinct; What does my intuition tell me?
> N = No/Not Now; What happens if I say "no?"

OVERALL

- What's my vision of an ideal labor and delivery?

- What can I do to optimize the chances of realizing my vision?

- What happens in the event that things don't go according to plan?

THE START OF LABOR

- What kind of environment will make me feel safe and calm for birth? (e.g., dim lights, minimal talking, use of words like "surges" instead of "contractions," staying positive, refraining from the word "pain," support for hypnobirthing, etc.)

- How can my partner or a support person help?

- What are my options with regard to vaginal exams? Do I want to keep track of my cervical dilation/effacement or do I want to be checked only when medically necessary? What about after my water breaks?

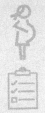

- How do I feel about being induced? How do I feel about the artificial rupture of membranes? What options do I have for no or low intervention?

- What are my options after my water breaks? What if there is meconium?

DURING LABOR

- How do I plan to manage sensations? What would I like to do if labor slows down? What are my preferences in case of a Cesarean?

- When do I want to move to the hospital or a birth center (if relevant)?

- If not at home, what would I like to be able to control in my physical environment? (e.g., temperature, lighting, sounds, smells, drinking and snacking, comfort measures, visitor management, etc.)

- What do I plan on doing to stay relaxed? (e.g., wear my own clothes, play certain kinds of music, use a birth ball and/or tub, etc.)

- What are the choices that affect my ability to move about freely? (e.g., how baby is monitored, medical interventions and medication, options for managing fluids, etc.)

- Do I want to be coached when it's time to push? If so, what kind of coaching is offered, and who do I want support from and in what way?

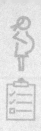

AFTER DELIVERING BABY

- What are my options with regard to cutting the umbilical cord? (e.g., immediate, delayed – for how long, lotus birth, etc.)

- What are the pros and cons of cord blood banking? How would choosing to do this affect my preferences related to cutting the umbilical cord?

- What are my options with circumcision if I have a baby boy? (e.g., leave uncircumcised, circumcise at facility upon delivery, circumcise at a later date and location)

- What are my options for delivering the placenta? (e.g., active versus physiological management of the third stage of labor)

- Upon delivery, what should I consider when deciding whether or not to keep the vernix? How long do I want to wait before giving baby a bath?

- How long would it be optimal for me to be able to hold baby undisturbed immediately after birth?

- What routine tests, shots, and/or medications are given for the baby in the first three days after birth? What options do we have?

- If breastfeeding is important to me, what will best support that? (e.g., immediate skin-to-skin contact, lactation consultant on call, delayed routine baby checks/bath/shots, withholding formula, rooming in, use of a hospital grade pump, etc.)

- Other potential considerations (e.g., placenta encapsulation, alternative newborn care and/or vaccination schedule, religious traditions, cultural customs, etc.)

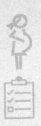

Chapter 20

SAMPLE
PARTNER SUPPORT PLAN

The best thing my husband and I did when preparing for delivery day was talk through our game plan (both at a high level and in detail) — how we hoped the birth would go and how he could best support me through labor, delivery, and in the first two weeks afterward (when he would be on parental leave). We went through the birth plan I had put together, what's driving my preferences, and the role I'd like him to play.

The following are some examples of how partners can support mamas-to-be . . .

AT HOME

- Deflecting phone calls and texts asking if baby is here yet
- Charging any devices (e.g., portable Bluetooth speakers, headphones) that may be needed at the hospital
- Helping her stay hydrated, nourished, relaxed, and as comfortable as possible in early labor
- Reminding her of comfort measures and providing hands-on support when needed (e.g., consider bookmarking

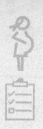

the *Sample Comfort Measures for Labor* chapter and/or creating a menu of your own)

- Reviewing the *Childbirth 101* chapter, keeping track of labor progress, and calling the provider with updates (e.g., recurring surges every 5–7 min, if water breaks, on the way to the hospital and ETA)

- Ensuring that the hospital bag is packed and the car seat is installed

AT THE HOSPITAL

- Being the primary person to interact with the care team

- Advocating for birth plan and preferences

- Taking pictures after baby is born and notifying family of the birth

- Asking questions related to postnatal and newborn care (and taking notes in this book)

AFTER BABY COMES HOME

- Supporting her rest and recovery (e.g., doing everything other than breastfeeding, encouraging mom to nap when the baby naps)

- Managing visitors and responding to offers for help (e.g., reminding guests to wash their hands, limiting visiting time to keep mom and baby from getting overtired, keeping a list of things that others can help with)

- Calling insurance to add baby to coverage (including additional phone calls to short-term disability and FMLA to confirm delivery date)

- Looking up answers to questions (related to the baby) first before asking mom and taking primary responsibility in calling for help when needed (e.g., pediatrician, lactation consultant, postpartum doula or night nurse, primary care provider)

While it's great to discuss your expectations for birth and for how things might go, remember that what happens will be largely out of your control. So be flexible, and have a mentality of rolling with the punches. This is just a precursor of what it'll soon be like to have an unpredictable baby. There's so much value in partners who stay relaxed and who model calmness during this time, as this will subconsciously help the birthing mother take your lead in staying as calm and relaxed as possible herself!

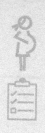

Chapter 21

FINDING A PEDIATRICIAN

QUESTIONS TO ASK A PROSPECTIVE PEDIATRICIAN (OR OFFICE SUPERVISOR)

1. **Do you accept my insurance? What's your new patient intake process if we selected you as our baby's pediatrician?**

2. **What are your hours?** (e.g., normal business hours, after-hours availability)
   - What is your protocol for after-hours support and care?
   - Where is your primary location? What other offices do you have, and what are the business hours for those locations?

3. **Who's available?**
   - Is it a physician group or an individual doctor?
   - Do we select a primary provider or do we see whomever is on call?
   - Who attends most of the appointments, a nurse practitioner or a pediatrician?
   - Are there lactation consultants on staff? What are their hours?

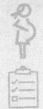

4. **What's your philosophy on the following?**
   - Vaccinations (including circumcision)
   - Breastfeeding versus formula-feeding
   - Co-sleeping and other parenting decisions related to baby care/sleep
   - Prescribing medication (e.g., for prevention versus treatment as needed)
   - Handling well-care versus sick care (including recommended well-care schedule for the baby's first year)

5. **What makes you stand out compared to other pediatricians?** (e.g., easy access to labs/imaging and other specialists, flexible vaccination schedule, 24/7 access to on-call physician, same-day sick appointments, on-site asthma clinic and/or vision care, easy access and seamless transfer of electronic health records, accepts walk-ins, flexible visitor policy, etc.)

6. **What other questions do you get from parents that would be helpful for me to know?**

Make sure you've made arrangements for a family physician or in-network pediatrician to be present at your baby's birth. This will help you avoid an expensive out-of-network bill from whomever is on call at the time of your delivery. Just because a hospital or birthing center is in-network doesn't guarantee that all of its staff are! And don't worry if you haven't yet found the perfect provider – you can always change later if needed.

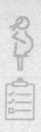

Chapter 22

SAMPLE PACKING LIST
FOR BIRTH DAY

Depending on where you choose to give birth, you may want to customize the list below. You may also find it useful to share your list with your providers to see if any of the items are not allowed in the facility, or if they have additional suggestions based on your birth plan.

FOR MOM

- Large bath towel
- Loose, comfy clothing (including sweatshirt in case room is cold)
- Bathing suit/swim skirt without crotch, shower shoes and grippy socks
- Travel toiletries (including chap stick, deodorant, glasses/contact lenses, brush/comb, hair ties, toothbrush)
- Pillow (regular and/or inflatable pillow for the tub)
- Massage tools and eye mask
- Aromatherapy (no candles)
- Warm pack/rice sock

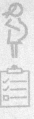

- Coconut water or caffeine-free electrolyte tablets for hydration
- Sugar-free lozenges for dry mouth during labor
- Garbage bags for laundry and old towels for car (in case water breaks)
- Come with nail polish removed (in case pulse oximeter is used)
- If breastfeeding: nursing pillow, robe, hands-free pumping bra and pump

FOR PARTNER

- Cell phones, headphones and chargers/battery packs
- Music player/portable Bluetooth speaker and charger
- IDs, insurance card and wallet
- Vitamins and/or medications/prescriptions (if applicable)
- Snacks (or coins for vending machines)
- Refillable water bottle
- Deodorant, glasses/contact lenses and change of clothing
- Swimsuit and shower shoes
- Five printed copies of your birth plan (including family physician or pediatrician info) and tape to put it up in your room
- Reading materials/audiobooks/podcasts, etc.
- This book! (including all your notes in the margins and any other loose pages stuffed into it)

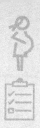

FOR BABY

- Rear-facing infant car seat
- Receiving blanket/swaddle
- Newborn onesie/sleeper
- Outfit/props for pictures
- Camera and charger
- Going home outfit with separated legs instead of gown if using car seat (including hat, mittens, and socks)
- If using cloth diapers and/or a particular kind of wipes is important to you, then you'll have to bring your own. Most hospitals will have plenty of disposable diapers and wipes on hand.

Consider packing separate bags for use during labor and after delivery. If parking is secure and easily accessible, it may be helpful to leave the post-delivery bag(s) in the trunk for later.

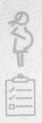

Chapter 23

SAMPLE COMFORT
MEASURES FOR LABOR

BREATHING AND MEDITATION

- Progressive relaxation: head to toe
- Close eyes, roll shoulders back, take a deep breath, bring attention to the sensation under your feet
- Calm and relaxed, out-breath is double the count of the in-breath (used during first stage of labor)
- Slow and focused, in- and out-breath are symmetrical like going up and down a hill (used during second stage of labor)
- Candle blowing (used during transition/during urge to push)

VISUALIZATION

- Favorite place to be together (e.g., warm, breezy, sandy beach; beautiful and fresh-smelling garden with soft patch of grass; lush mountainside with a breathtaking view for miles)
- Print out a picture and put it up in the room to have a focal point

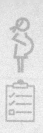

- Air balloon rising with a beautiful sunrise (can be used during labor as a metaphor for the uterus contracting upward and cervix relaxing open)
- Soft ripples slowly drifting outward in a serene lake (can be used during labor as a metaphor for the baby moving down the birth canal)
- Positive affirmations and mantras (e.g., "open and soften")

TOOLS AND ENVIRONMENT

- Battery-operated fan
- Heat/cold packs (e.g., rice socks)
- Music
- Aromatherapy/diffuser/candles
- Water: shower, tub
- Peaceful/dimly lit room
- Massage tools
- Peanut and/or birthing ball

TOUCH

- Massage: light touch, firm stroke, deep massage
- Use hands to massage body, with or without lotion
- Counter pressure/hip squeeze

MOVEMENT

- Relax the jaw to relax the pelvic region
- Squatting positions using a birth ball (rocking and swaying)
- Side lunges (foot can be placed on a bed or chair)
- Walking
- Slow dancing, moving hips in a circular motion to open the pelvis

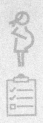

Chapter 24

CHILDBIRTH 101

1ˢᵗ Stage of Labor: Thinning and Opening of the Cervix (you may want to have your partner download in advance a free timer app like the Full Term Contraction Timer for iOS mobile)

- **Early labor** (e.g., irregular duration of contractions, spaced 20–30 min apart, 0–6 cm dilated): just relax during this time and stay home; can last 6–12+ hrs

- **Active labor** (e.g., 45 sec duration of contractions, spaced 2–3 min apart, 6–8 cm dilated): stay focused, upright and calm; keep moving and allow gravity to help; can last 3–5 hrs

- **Transition** (e.g., 60–90 sec duration of contractions, spaced closely together, 8–10 cm dilated): breathe deeply to give your baby plenty of oxygen; this is the hardest but shortest, but you are strong and you can do it; can last 30 min to 2 hrs

2ⁿᵈ Stage of Labor: Pushing and Birth

- Commences when 10 cm dilated; if unmedicated, will feel overwhelming urge similar to a bowel movement; go with your instincts and trust your body to breathe the baby down; can last 20 min to 2 hrs (for first-time moms)

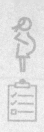

3rd Stage of Labor: Delivery of the Placenta

- Oxytocin generated from holding the baby skin-to-skin will naturally trigger the placenta to detach and expel from the body; can happen 5–20 min after birth

- Personal choice of physiological versus active management of the third stage of labor – do your own independent research and then have a conversation with your health care provider (If your wishes differ from the "standard protocol/policy," ask for their recommendation in writing and/or if you can sign a waiver to support your decision.)

4th Stage of Labor: Recovery and Bonding

- Mild contractions may occur as the uterus starts to return to its regular size (this may be aided by breastfeeding within the first hour of birth); some bleeding may occur

- If breastfeeding is important to you: ask if rooming-in with your baby is possible; ask if a lactation consultant or nurse is available to help

Depending on your provider, you may be given choices that are presented as matter-of-fact or as strong recommendations. Remember that you always have a choice, and to use B.R.A.I.N. (benefits, risks, alternatives, intuition and instinct, no/not now) to evaluate what's right for you. For example, many women accept epidurals without knowing that it can slow down labor, or that contractions with Pitocin are harder, stronger, and peak faster. As long as you are aware of the full range of options (and their implications) at your disposal, you'll hopefully be able to minimize negative surprises.

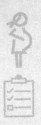

Chapter 25

WHY ISN'T BABY HERE YET?

Your bags are packed, you're all stocked up on diapers and a changing pad and onesies, you're mentally prepared (as well as you can be), your friends and family (and coworkers and seemingly strangers on the street) are asking you for a daily update. Your due date has come and gone. And baby is still. Not. Here.

Did you know that due dates vary by country and by method of calculation? (The best dating method is with a first trimester ultrasound.) Regardless of how you measure it, 80% of people deliver between weeks 38 and 42. The average for low-risk, first-time moms is closer to 41 weeks if calculating from the start of the last menstrual period. This is all to say – don't freak out! If the non-stress tests, ultrasounds, and all else point to a healthy fetus, then know that you are doing just fine, mama! Don't fret – baby will come at the perfect time precisely when he or she is ready.

BUT . . . (and I can hear you now as you're still not convinced) "Is there anything natural I can do to help baby come out sooner?" Well, yes and no. No in that there's no real evidence that says if you do xyz, then baby will come the next day. HOWEVER. Yes, there are things that have anecdotally contributed to encouraging cervical ripeness and to stimulating the onset of labor. These aren't surefire methods, but if

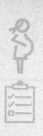

they give you a sense of feeling more in control of the situation by taking every natural action possible, then below are some ideas to encourage the spontaneous start of labor: (Be sure to discuss first with your health care provider to ensure there are no contraindications for you, especially if you have gestational diabetes or high blood pressure.)

PHYSICAL ENCOURAGEMENT

- Walk. A lot. Like 1–2 hours a day if the thought of doing so doesn't wear you out.

- Do squats. Do lunges. Sit on an exercise ball and bounce on it. Be gentle!

- Have sex. They say that the prostaglandins in sperm help to ripen the cervix.

- Stimulate your nipples. If using a breast pump, then it's best to do so under the watch of your health care provider so as to not risk stressing the baby.

- Acupuncture and/or acupressure with a certified professional who knows what they're doing.

ENVIRONMENTAL ENCOURAGEMENT

- Diffuse clary sage and jasmine essential oils.

- Mix clary sage essential oil with a carrier oil or lotion and rub on your belly.

- Reduce stress and try to relax as much as you can. If you haven't been already, now is the time to pamper yourself!

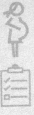

NUTRITIONAL ENCOURAGEMENT

- Eat spicy food.

- Eat pineapple.

- Drink red raspberry leaf tea.

- Eat 6 dates a day.

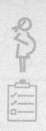

Chapter 26

SAMPLE BIRTH AFFIRMATIONS

Regardless of what is in your birth plan, it can be greatly beneficial to amass a list of quotes, affirmations, and other inspiration to help you build and sustain confidence during pregnancy and labor. Below are two questions and sample affirmations to help you build your list.

1. WHY IS MY VISION IMPORTANT TO ME?

Normal women's bodies are able to handle the sensations that arise naturally during childbirth.

Assume I am normal and that my body will behave normally. I am built to be able to handle the natural sensations and hormones my body produces during labor.

By avoiding (or delaying) any intervention of any kind, I'm not only avoiding the introduction of risk to a natural process, but I'm also giving myself and my baby the best chances of a quicker, easier recovery following birth. (e.g., no adverse effects from medication or on breastfeeding, less chance of perineal tearing if no epidural, reduced risk of emergency C-section if no

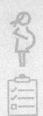

induction, increased ability to handle contractions if no induction, no risk of baby being drowsy from medications if none given during labor, reduced risk of episiotomy or having to use vacuum/forceps if no epidural, etc.)

By delaying going to the hospital as long as possible during early labor, I prolong the amount of time that I can be in the comfort of my own home.

2. HOW CAN I ACHIEVE MY VISION?

During pregnancy:

- Getting in the best shape possible through healthy eating, regular exercise, and practicing mental and emotional self-care will help me and my baby.

- I am surrounding myself with any and all resources to sustain my vision and my *why*. (e.g., childbirth education classes – online or in person; hearing or reading about birth stories similar to the type of birth you'd like to have; practicing hypnobirthing, meditation, visualization and/or breathing exercises such that they become second nature)

During labor and delivery:

- I can let go of my inhibitions. I can make the noises I'm called to make. I can allow my body to be how it will be. There's nothing I can do that my health care providers haven't seen before. I will get into my flow and go with it.

- I am very present. I am closing my eyes, and my partner will shut the blinds and turn off the lights if it helps. I

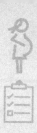

only need to just focus on the current surge and breathe through it. (As a marathon runner, the analogy that resonated with me was just looking to get to the next mile marker – e.g., the next surge, or the next centimeter of dilation – instead of thinking about finishing the race – e.g., delivering the baby.)

- Transition is the hardest part. Once I get through that, my body will give me the recovery I need between surges.

- I can do it! It is possible. Women have been doing this for hundreds of thousands of years. I can do it too. My body was made to do it. I am strong and capable.

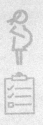

Chapter 27

ASSEMBLING
KEY INFO AND CONTACTS

Prior to giving birth, it helps to have all of your key contacts, passwords, and notes about what you (or your partner) need to do all in one place. Feel free to write it directly in this chapter and/or staple a notecard to this page.

Health care providers: (e.g., phone number, email if provided, fax, address, business hours, after-hours/emergency/nursing support/mental health support line, telehealth details including login info)

- Family physician and/or pediatrician

- Lactation consultant

- Mom's primary care physician, therapist, and/or other provider(s)

Miscellaneous: (e.g., phone number, email if provided, address, business hours, after-hours line)

- Emergency contacts (at least one local)

- Local police non-emergency line

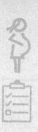

- Essential coworkers (e.g., boss, HR/staffing manager)

- Health insurance and/or HR benefits center (depending on your employer, this may be one phone number with automated prompts or separate phone numbers for each type of benefit): general inquiries, short-term disability, FMLA

- Doula, night nurse, sleep consultant, and/or other hired help

Info your insurance company and/or HR benefits center may need from you:

- Adding baby to coverage: phone, group/subscriber number, baby's full name and DOB

- Use of short-term disability (for mom) and/or FMLA leave (for either parent): phone number, claim/request number, employer and employee ID, baby's DOB

Make sure to write down login details for non-confidential accounts and mobile apps, especially if sharing an account for use on several devices. (e.g., smart home, baby tracker apps, SNOO, Hatch, etc.) You definitely don't want to be in a position of having to reset an account password at 3am while handling a fussy infant!

POSTNATAL

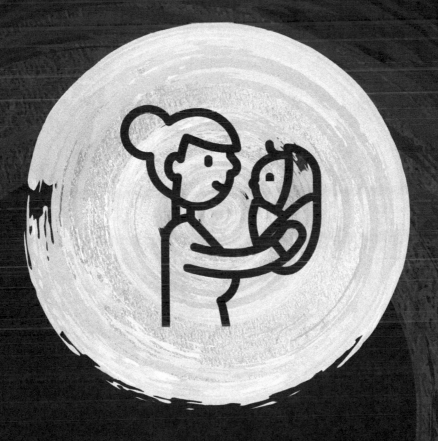

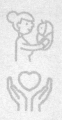

Chapter 28

GIVING YOURSELF GRACE

You've finally made it past labor and delivery, woohoo! For many, the birth itself can feel like a marathon effort. You've prepared yourself for that moment for nine months (sometimes more), and now that baby is finally here, it can feel a bit chaotic simply because now there is no clear "finish line."

If I had to pick one chapter in this whole book that you should bookmark and come back to time and again in that first year of motherhood, this would be the one. As a new parent, your attention will be pulled in a million directions. What even constitutes success during this time? From a whole health standpoint, it takes plenty of effort just to stay sane, be nourished, and enjoy this roller coaster of a journey into a new chapter in your life.

"When you take time to replenish your spirit, it allows you to serve others from the overflow. You cannot serve from an empty vessel." —Eleanor Brown

During this hormone-filled postnatal period, it can often be difficult to get out of your own head. The following is wisdom that many moms have shared with me. On the right is a list of common anxieties. On the left are perspectives that came over time. Whenever you feel tempted to doubt yourself, come back

PART IV

POSTNATAL SELF-CARE

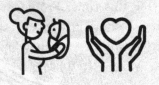

to this list and add your worry, then write next to it what you'll say, do, or think instead.

SAY THIS...	NOT THAT...
"Thanks so much for offering to help. Here's what we need most right now . . ."	"What will they think of me if I ask for help?"
"I won't be available for at least another month or two. I underestimated what having a baby would mean. Hope you will understand."	"I have to live up to every promise."
"I can make time for what's most important. Chores can wait. Writing notes and answering the phone can be done later. Nothing sounds better right now than taking a nap."	"I never have time for anything."
"For my own and my baby's sake, it's imperative that I continually check in on my physical, mental, and emotional needs."	"I can take care of myself later."
"I am letting go of my need to always be in control. I recognize my need to take a break, and I am giving myself permission to do so."	"My baby needs me for everything. No one else can do it like I can."
"I've left my baby in good hands, and I have a choice to be anxious or not while I'm gone."	"I can't take any time away from baby. What if something goes wrong?"
"I don't need to get anything done right now. It's OK to just rest, recover, and be present with my child."	"I can't get anything done."

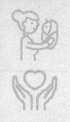

Chapter 29

UPPING YOUR MENTAL GAME

Nobody ever said parenthood is easy. But that doesn't mean you should let yourself wallow in self-pity and focus on how hard it is. As any athlete or performer can attest, the talk track in our heads can either make or break us in practice and in competition (or on stage). Often things don't go according to plan, and conditions may be unfavorable.

"Whether you think you can or you think you can't, you're right." —Henry Ford

BE WITH WHAT IS

Things are as they are and you can be with them as they are.

- You are resilient.
- You have strength.
- You can handle it.

KEEP GOING

This, too, shall pass.

- You have control over what you think – don't let your inner thoughts beat you up.

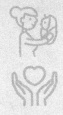

- You are not your thoughts – step back and let your thoughts pass like clouds.

- The first 100 days are the hardest. It *will* get easier.

VISUALIZE SUCCESS

Be specific about what you want and why you want it.

- You are not defined by your role.

- You are multifaceted.

- You are able to define your own identity (so that others don't do it for you).

LEARN AND GROW

Embrace the opportunity.

- What can you learn from this?

- How can you grow from this?

- What do you have to gain from all of this?

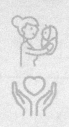

Chapter 30

NUTRITION AND NOURISHMENT

Always, always, always **have a bottle of water within hand's reach**. Staying hydrated (just aim for clear urine rather than counting how many glasses you're drinking) can really help to reduce fatigue, increase energy, and alleviate headaches and muscle cramps. Not to mention, having plenty of fluids (e.g., coconut water, soups, electrolytes) can greatly help in preventing clogged ducts if breastfeeding.

Consume a balanced diet. Keep up the healthy eating habits you maintained throughout pregnancy! This will do wonders for your physical and mental well-being, and will also be critical for baby if you choose to breastfeed. Keep taking your prenatal vitamins. Ask your provider if you also need to consider supplementing with vitamin D, B12, and/or gentle iron. Note that it may be worth speaking with a family physician, pediatrician, and/or a lactation consultant about potential foods to avoid if breastfeeding (e.g., dairy, peppermint, sage, caffeine, alcohol).

Stock up on healthy snacks. (e.g., fresh fruit, mini cucumbers, pre-cut veggies and hummus, low sodium popcorn, unsweetened granola, ready-made quinoa salad, etc.) Have meals in the freezer, your favorite smoothie recipes on hand, and grocery/

food delivery apps downloaded. Consider also having your partner work out a schedule (e.g., manually or via a shared Google doc) for when family and friends who've offered to help can drop off homemade meals.

Don't weigh yourself. No need to put a time limit on "bouncing back." Your body just did a miraculous and incredible thing – you just birthed a living, breathing human being! Try to be patient with your body and with your mind. No one is judging you on what you look like – honestly, we're all just in awe that you're somehow able to care for another person while managing to keep yourself alive at the same time! You truly are amazing, mama!

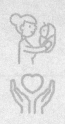

Chapter 31

PHYSICAL RECOVERY
FROM BIRTH

A mom's body changes throughout pregnancy and goes through a lot during birth. After baby is born, the body continues to go through changes, commonly in the following ways . . .

SHRINKING OF THE UTERUS
BACK TO ITS ORIGINAL SIZE

What may occur:

- Afterpains in the uterus (especially while breastfeeding)
- Vaginal bleeding (lochia) with color gradually changing from red to brown to white

What may help:

- Use breathing techniques to relax during afterpains
- Wear pads (instead of tampons) to reduce the risk of infection

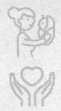

SORENESS IN THE PELVIC FLOOR (FOR VAGINAL BIRTHS)

What may occur:

- Soreness in the perineum and pelvic floor for several weeks postpartum

What may help:

- Apply ice packs in the first 24 hrs after birth
- Run warm water over the area while in the shower
- Take a warm bath or sitz bath (that fits on the toilet)
- Use witch hazel pads or a numbing spray
- Ask your provider about the best way to approach
- Kegel exercises to increase circulation
- Avoid using tampons

BREAST MILK PRODUCTION

What may occur:

- First milk is clear, thick, golden fluid called colostrum (which increases and changes to mature milk within a few days)
- Newborns lose 7–10% of their birth weight within the first two weeks

What may help (if choosing to breastfeed):

- Breastfeed often (the more baby eats, the more milk the body will produce) – newborns need to be breast-fed 8–12 times every 24 hrs (including at least 1–2 night feedings until they surpass their birth weight)

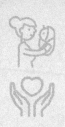

- Wake baby if it's been more than 4 hrs since the last feeding

- Let baby breastfeed as long as there is active sucking and swallowing

- Switch breasts for each feeding (it will usually feel fuller)

- Try to feed baby before he/she cries

- Avoid pacifiers until breastfeeding is going well and milk production is established

- Use pillows for support and hold baby close to body

- Re-latch if baby only has the nipple or a small amount of breast in his/her mouth – don't put up with nipple pain or soreness

- Hand express or pump milk if experiencing uncomfortable fullness or engorgement

- To prevent clogged ducts, remove milk regularly from both breasts, wear loose clothing, avoid sleeping on stomach, use a hospital grade breast pump, gently massage the breasts, and/or ask your healthcare provider about the use of sunflower lecithin

- Consult your provider immediately if you experience breast pain, swelling, warmth, fever, and chills

- See a lactation consultant for personal guidance (this is helpful for all new moms, but especially if you haven't started producing milk within a few days after delivery)

What may help (to recognize feeding cues):

- Baby opens mouth, sticks tongue out, makes sucking movements/sounds, brings hand to mouth, moves legs (like crawling), turns toward the breast

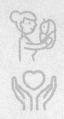

Chapter 32

BODY AFTER BABY

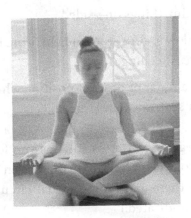

FIRST, BREATHE.

Breathe from the diaphragm.

Think of breath and proper posture with all movements. (e.g., sitting to standing, lifting, bending) Remember to exhale on the exertion!

Head-to-Toe Posture Tips:

- Align the *cervical spine* and reduce *neck* pain (by releasing and strengthening the neck)
- Reverse rounded *shoulders* (by opening the chest and strengthening the muscles between the shoulder blades)
- Reduce *low back* pain and reverse lumbar lordosis (by stretching the lumbar muscles and strengthening the ab corset)

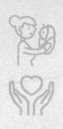

- Align the *pelvis* and *hips* (by picturing a bowl formed by the bones around the pelvis, and keeping the contents in the bowl from spilling over)

- Improve circulation and prevent *leg* cramps (by stretching and foam rolling the legs and feet)

- Avoid doing things one-sided

- Use a pillow and/or stool to help bring baby to you while breastfeeding

- Assume a squat or deadlift position when lifting the baby, car seat, or other large objects

Recommence Kegel exercises as soon as you feel comfortable. (Ask a provider to explain how to do them even if you think you know. Note that there may be individual circumstances when Kegels are contraindicated.)

SECOND, WALK SLOWLY.

Rest before you think you might need to – start small and build up gradually.

If you notice heavier bleeding, then back off – don't hesitate to call your health care provider if you have any questions.

Consult the American College of Obstetricians and Gynecologists (ACOG) and the American Council on Exercise (ACE) for exercise guidance in the prenatal and postpartum period.

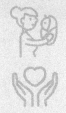

FINALLY, BE PLANFUL, AND SEEK PROFESSIONAL SUPPORT AND GUIDANCE.

Consider all aspects of your physical fitness – balance, flexibility, cardio, and strength.

Check out perinatal functional fitness and women's health physical therapy.

- Some examples of what these professionals can help with include: back pain, incontinence, pelvic rehab, pelvic core dysfunction, diastasis recti, pain during or after sex, carpal tunnel, and more.

- Call your insurance company to check if you're covered!

- What may be seen as just another optional preventive measure in the U.S. is considered routine care in other countries, especially if you are recovering from a C-section.

Look into massage therapy, chiropractic care, and/or acupuncture (with clearance from your health care provider).

Ease into personal training, mom and baby fitness classes, and/or specialized postnatal programs.

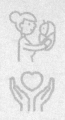

Chapter 33

HOW PARTNERS CAN HELP

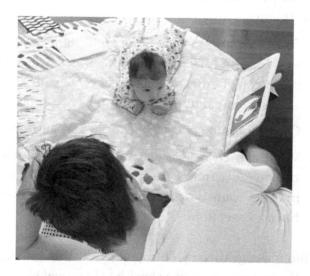

Just because a partner can't breastfeed doesn't mean he or she can't bond with the baby. Here are some ideas for partners who want to be more involved:

- Get mom something to drink or eat while she is nursing (and ensure that water is always within reaching distance)

- Help keep baby awake during feedings by rubbing feet or stroking hands/legs

- Give mom a shoulder rub (especially during or after breastfeeding)

- Give baby a massage (if baby is calm and/or in a good mood)

- Take over childcare between feedings so mom can get some rest or have some time to herself

- Take over the household chores and/or be the one responsible for figuring out how they get done

- Make eye contact with baby (newborns can focus on objects that are 8–14 inches away – they like to look at human faces and bold, contrasting shapes and colors)

- Hold baby close (newborns can feel temperature, texture, pressure, and pain – they love to feel your skin, so continue to hold your newborn skin-to-skin at home)

- Talk to your baby – newborns can hear well and are able to tell the difference between a range of sounds, including the voices of their parents (e.g., take a tour of the house and talk about what they're looking at; label feelings and narrate what they're doing; ask them what they see, where they're going, etc.)

- Take baby for a walk

- Rock, cuddle, play with, bathe, change, read and sing to, and burp the baby

- Sensory play – engage the baby's different senses (e.g., taste, touch, smell, hearing, sight, vestibular or awareness of body balance/movement, proprioceptive or sense of body position)

- Go with mom to sick visits and well-baby checkups

- Take an infant CPR/first aid class

- Learn how to soothe the baby with the 5 S's (swaddle, side/stomach position, shush, swing, suck)

- Take candid photos of mom and baby

- Tell mom she is doing an amazing job and that you're so proud of her!

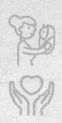

Don't forget to take care of yourself too during this time!

- Eat well and exercise

- Sleep or rest as much as you can

- Find other new parents you can talk to

- Pay attention to your emotions (partners can get depressed too)

Watch for post-birth warning signs *(see the next 2 chapters)*

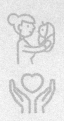

Chapter 34

LIFESAVING WARNING SIGNS: MOM

Most moms who give birth recover without problems. But <u>any</u> mom can have complications after the birth of a baby. Learning to recognize these post-birth warning signs (and enlisting your partner to also learn them) can save your life. Pending your specific situation, discuss with your provider other potential signs to watch for.

Call 9-1-1 or go to the ER if you have:

- Pain in chest, obstructed breathing, or shortness of breath (may mean you have a blood clot in your lung or a heart problem)

- Seizures (may mean you have a condition called eclampsia)

- Thoughts of hurting self or baby (may mean you have postpartum depression)

Call your health care provider if you have:
- Heavy bleeding, soaking through 1 pad/hr, blood clots larger than a golf ball (may mean you have an obstetric hemorrhage)

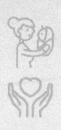

- Incision that isn't healing, increased redness or any pus from episiotomy or C-section site (may mean you have an infection)

- Red or swollen leg that is painful or warm to touch (may mean you have a blood clot)

- Temperature of 100.4 degrees F or higher, foul smelling vaginal blood or discharge (may mean you have an infection)

- Headache that doesn't get better, even after taking medicine, or bad headache with vision changes (may mean you have high blood pressure or post birth preeclampsia)

- Severe pain in your lower belly or increased uterine pain (may mean you have endometriosis, which is inflammation in the lining of the uterus)

- Pain or burning with urination, pain in the lower back/side or needing to pee often (may mean you have a urinary tract infection)

- Lump, hard area, redness, or pain in your breast (may mean you have a clogged duct or mastitis)

If you aren't able to get ahold of your health care provider, then call 9-1-1 or go to the ER. Don't delay getting medical care!

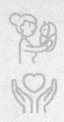

Chapter 35
Lifesaving Warning Signs: Baby

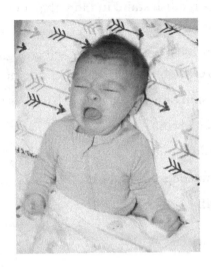

Call 9-1-1 or go to the ER, whichever is faster, if baby has:

- Lips, tongue, or mouth are blue
- Serious difficulty breathing

Call your family physician or pediatrician if baby has the following signs of illness:

- Refusing to eat or not eating well (for newborns, this could look like: difficulty latching on, frequently goes longer than 4 hrs between feedings, frequently needs to be awakened to feed, has not regained birth weight within 10–14 days, often acts hungry after breastfeeding, has fewer than 6 wet diapers and 4 dirty diapers by day 5, sleeps through the night, a drastic change in stool patterns after the first week)

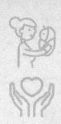

- Stools that look like pebbles (may mean baby has constipation)

- Watery stools (may mean baby has diarrhea); white stools or stools with blood or mucus

- Urate (a reddish stain) in more than one diaper after the first 72 hrs

- Fever of 100.4 degrees Fahrenheit or higher (or about 99 degrees Fahrenheit if taken under the arm)

- Yellow skin or eyes (may mean baby has jaundice)

- Constant crying

- Projectile vomiting

- Frequent coughing and/or difficulty breathing

- Pale skin

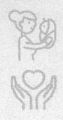

Chapter 36

FIVE STEPS
TO FIGHTING OVERWHELM

This is a short exercise to help you take a step back and organize your thoughts when feeling stressed and/or overwhelmed. Ideally, you're able to set aside 15–20 minutes. But if you only have five minutes, then spend five minutes now and come back to it later. However much time you choose, make sure you set a timer – that will help to focus your thoughts.

STEP 1: Get out a sheet of paper and brain dump anything and everything onto the page. Get it all out. Bullet points encouraged. This could include, but is not limited to, feelings, to do's, worries, reminders, questions, etc. Typing it out on your phone or laptop works too if that's handy.

STEP 2: Once you've got a good list, go through each item and mark the ones that would help you the most if resolved first. Don't get bogged down by the "how" just yet.

STEP 3: Pick <u>one</u> of the items you marked. To help you choose, ask yourself, "What's the smallest thing I can tackle now that will have the biggest impact?"

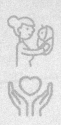

STEP 4: For that one thing you picked, what would need to happen so that it no longer bothers you or takes up mental space? Who or what resources do you have at your disposal to help?

STEP 5: Go back to your brain dump and cross it off the list.

Revisit this exercise as often as needed, either individually or with your partner until you start feeling better.

PART V

POSTNATAL CRUCIAL CONVERSATIONS

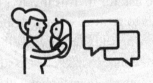

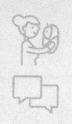

Chapter 37

SETTING BOUNDARIES

"Figure out what you want and learn how to ask for it." That's something I say often to myself and my coaching clients. Let me break it down:

> **Figure out what you want.** This means reflecting on what's important to you, trying things, letting go of perfection, and expecting to fail so you can learn from it. For new moms, this is especially important because it can be very unsettling to feel like you don't know what you don't know.

> **Learn how to ask for it.** This involves gaining the knowledge and skills to go after what you *do* want. A big part of this is also having the humility to admit what you don't know, the confidence to ask for help, and the discipline to persevere through challenges that will inevitably arise.

While this can serve as a life motto, it can also be directly applicable whenever there is uncertainty about how you should proceed. Setting boundaries is a perfect example.

Under normal circumstances, it can be hard for us to know what to do or how to respond to people who push up against our boundaries. It can be even more challenging during the

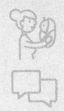

postpartum period (especially during flu season, or, as was the case when I wrote this book, in the midst of a global pandemic). If you feel yourself paralyzed with fear and anxiety about how to tell your loved ones "no" – follow these 5 steps for a better outcome for everyone involved:

1. **Figure out what your boundaries are** (e.g., What is and is not ok with you? When/under what circumstances? With whom?)

2. **Inform the other person** that they have violated your boundaries (e.g., "When you do __, it makes me feel __.")

3. **Ask for the new behavior you desire** and be specific (e.g., "In the future when __ happens, I ask that you please __ instead.")

4. **State the consequences** if your boundaries are not respected (e.g., "If you do __, then I will __." "If you don't do __, then I will __.")

5. **Enforce the consequences** (e.g., "It's not acceptable to me that __. I'm open to discussing this with you at a later time if you are interested, but right now, I must stand by my boundaries and __.")

Sample boundaries statements to use with well-meaning family and friends:

- "Appreciate you thinking of us! We'll definitely let you know when we're open to having people over."

- "We are enjoying this new and exciting time to bond as a family. Can't wait to catch up when things settle down!"

- "Really looking forward to seeing you! Just a heads-up, we're asking all visitors to wash their hands and wear a mask while at our house."

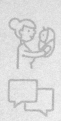

- "Thank you so much for making dinner. If you could send a text when you get here, we can visit from the doorway or through the window."

- "No, that doesn't work for us. We're not comfortable with that right now."

- "Thanks for your concern and input. We'll take time to consider all the options and decide what is best for our family."

- "Thanks for thinking of us. Unfortunately, we won't be able to make it to __. Enjoy/congrats!"

- "This is what we're doing for now, but it may change."

Remember that under __no__ circumstance are you required to say WHY you have the boundaries you've set. Your boundaries are what they are, and you never need to defend yourself for having them.

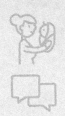

Chapter 38

SAMPLE DIVISION OF RESPONSIBILITIES

Taking care of a baby is hard. The longer your partner has time off from work to help you, the better. In the beginning, it can feel crazy and unsustainable even when both parents are home. It gets even harder when the partner must return to work.

If by now, you're feeling resentful, don't worry. This is actually fairly normal. After all, the mom is the one who had to carry the child, give birth, deal with so many hormonal changes, and if breastfeeding, take on what feels like a whole new full-time job. Don't feel bad or like a nag if you ask your partner (and others) constantly for help. Partners are not mind readers, so the more you share that you'd like for them to volunteer to take on certain things, the higher the likelihood they do help with those things! Take comfort that it will not be this hard forever. That's worth repeating. Keep reminding yourself that it will not always be this hard. For most, the first 100 days are the toughest, so know that there is indeed light at the end of the tunnel.

Our baby came during COVID-19, which meant that we weren't able to rely on family for the first six months. The silver lining for us, though, was the unexpected ability to work remotely brought on by the global pandemic. By the end of the first

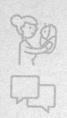

month, our division of labor settled loosely into me taking the "day shift" and my husband being on "night watch." By defining responsibilities and staying in dialogue about what was working (or not), we were equipped to manage stressful situations later when we were both tired and the baby was crying.

MOM

- 8am–5:30pm, everything baby needs, Mon–Fri (9.5 active hrs/day)
- 5am + 8pm pumping + 11pm feeding and put back to bed (1.5 active hrs/day)
- Prepare and wash bottles
- Grocery/pantry/restaurant orders
- Replenish baby supplies

PARTNER

- 5:30–11pm and 11:30pm–8am, everything baby needs, including bedtime routine and bathing, Mon–Fri (4.5 active hrs/day)
- Ad hoc time during the workday for breaks to relieve mom
- Baby's laundry 2x/wk
- Empty diaper pail 2x/wk
- House cleaning ad hoc
- Water all plants 2x/wk
- Collect trash and take out garbage and recycling
- Manage all dishwashing
- Manage budget

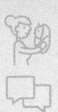

JOINT

- Meal prep
- Laundry
- Weekend time alone and with baby
- Printed weekly checklist of household chores (partner has primary responsibility, but mom to help when possible)
- Weekly check-in conversation to discuss what's working well (or not) and how to help each other

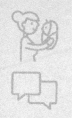

Chapter 39

COMMON EMOTIONAL CHANGES: MOM

CHANGES TO EXPECT AFTER BIRTH

- Some moms "fall in love" with baby immediately; others need a period of time to get acquainted before they feel a strong bond – both are normal

- Disappointment or anger with pregnancy, labor, delivery, and/or fussy baby

- Discomfort or irritability as a result of dealing with physical recovery

- Extreme fatigue or exhaustion from lack of sleep and/or anxiety about baby

- Tears at the drop of a hat due to decreased hormone levels after birth

- Baby blues during the first 2–3 wks after birth (usually intermittent and short-lived)

- Anxiety related to a postpartum body that looks and feels different or adjusting to the new role of mother and parent

- Jealousy or disappointment with others' focus and attention on the baby

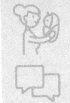

- Loss of control, feeling of being overwhelmed, anxious, or inadequate with baby's intense dependency and needs

- Resentment or anger toward partner who has no physical recovery and can seemingly return to pre-baby routines while leaving mom alone to take care of baby

- Feelings of isolation because of spending so much time with baby and no time with other adults

- Mixed feelings about intimacy with partner (e.g., physically not ready but wants to stay connected to partner)

WHAT MAY HELP

- Sleep (or at least try to nap) when baby sleeps

- Turn off the phone and resist the urge to constantly check email and/or social media

- Focus on rest and recovery in the first month after birth – let others worry about the housework and anything else that pops up

- Attend a weekly new mom's support group

- Schedule play dates with other moms and babies or with a close friend

- Plan a weekly date night with your partner where you spend time focused on each other

- Lower your expectations for yourself (especially regarding what your house looks like or your personal appearance)

- Get out of the house every day, even if it's just for 10 min, even if it's just to take a walk around the block; get some fresh air and take some deep breaths; best if you get out to pamper yourself (e.g., massage, mani/pedi)

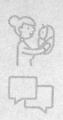

- Don't hesitate to seek help from family, friends, or health professionals – feel free to delegate to your partner the responsibility of accepting help when others offer

- Share this page with your partner and discuss how you can help each other

Remember that when the going gets hard, keep going. It's hardest in the beginning, and things will get easier. Try to focus on the positive and give your partner grace as much as you can.

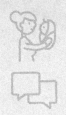

Chapter 40

COMMON EMOTIONAL CHANGES: PARTNER

CHANGES TO EXPECT AFTER BIRTH

- Anxiety, loss of control, or isolation (especially if the partner becomes the primary caregiver for baby while mom returns to work)

- Helplessness, jealousy, or feeling left out as the baby seemingly takes up all of mom's time and energy

- Feeling inadequate or clueless about taking care of baby while maternal instincts make mom seem like a natural with baby

- Increased stress and feeling the weight of responsibility to provide for the whole family and be a good parent

- Mixed feelings about intimacy (e.g., wants partner to feel comfortable but also wants to be physically connected)

- Feeling uncertain about how to deal with baby blues or postpartum mood disorders

WHAT MAY HELP

- Take ownership of some part of your baby's care (e.g., bath, burping, diaper changes, etc.) and take turns getting a stretch of uninterrupted sleep at night

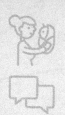

- Initiate back rubs/hugs/physical touch and give compliments without expecting anything else

- Don't hesitate to seek help from family, friends, or health professionals – take responsibility for sharing how others can help and accepting the help they offer

- Take the lead in arranging a weekly date night with your partner where you spend time focused on each other

- Pay attention to how your partner is handling things and call for help if you suspect a perinatal mood disorder

- Remember that this too shall pass – when the going gets hard, keep going

- It's hardest in the beginning – things <u>will</u> get easier

> Try to focus on the positive and take really good care of your partner. Treat each other with grace, don't take things personally, and keep an open dialogue about your feelings.

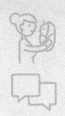

Chapter 41

POSTNATAL AND NEWBORN CARE: THE 10 B'S

Here are the key questions and topics to consider discussing with your provider(s) in the first few days and weeks after delivery . . .

1. BABY

- When to expect health assessments, well-care visits, and immunizations (e.g., within 2 days of birth, 1 week, 1 / 2 / 4 / 6 / 9 / 12 months, etc.),

- What to watch out for (e.g., signs of jaundice, ear infections) and what common things parents tend to call about in the first few weeks

- Guidance for general hygiene, umbilical cord/circumcision care, feeding cadence and volume, growth and weight gain (including expected return to birth weight)

- Preventive measures to reduce chance of ear infections (e.g., breastfeeding for 3–6 months, avoid second-hand smoke exposure, have baby sit upright while drinking from the bottle)

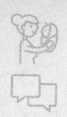

2. BREASTS

- Milk supply and production, collection and storage
- Latch and/or positioning of baby, nipple care, preventing clogged ducts and treating mastitis
- Any dietary supplements the birthing mother should take (e.g., prenatal vitamin, iron, vitamin D)
- Resources and lactation consultant/nursing services (including how and when a hospital grade breast pump may be used)

3. BOWELS

- How to prevent or treat constipation to reduce perineal pain (e.g., high fiber diet, increased water intake)
- When to expect resolution of incontinence (e.g., 3 months)

4. BLADDER

- When and how often to do Kegel exercises (e.g., resume after 3 weeks, any contraindications)
- When to expect resolution of urinary symptoms (e.g., 3 months), including when referrals may be needed for pelvic floor physiotherapist/urogynecologist

5. BELLY

- How to assess and treat pain
- What to watch out for (including when to see a provider)

PART VI

POSTNATAL CHECKLIST

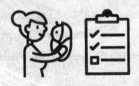

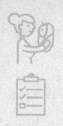

Chapter 42

THE CHECKLIST: POSTNATAL

- **Prioritize the mother's rest and recovery** (including drinking plenty of water and maintaining a nutritious diet) – you have to put the oxygen mask on yourself before you're able to take care of anyone else!

- Ask hospital staff about their standard protocol for getting your baby's **birth certificate** and **social security number**

- **Call insurance to add baby to coverage** (including following up with FMLA and/or short-term disability to update them on your delivery date) – **If breastfeeding**, ask your provider or pediatrician for a referral to a **lactation consultant** sooner rather than later to ensure proper latching and optimal use of a hospital grade pump to build and establish milk supply

- **Disable doorbell** (or put up a sign) to minimize disturbances when baby is sleeping

- Bring a list of questions you have for the **baby's first doctor's appointment** (feel free to leverage the 10 B's in the previous chapter)

- **Love on your baby!** Make eye contact, talk to, play with, and interact with your newborn – pay attention to your baby's cries and start to gain an understanding of what he/she is trying to communicate

- Establish a cadence of checking in with your partner on a regular basis about your physical, mental, and emotional needs – you'll both need self-care, and having a regular conversation about it can be helpful to remind you both to keep an open dialogue on this very important aspect of parenting!

- **Notify loved ones** about the wonderful new addition to your family

- **Get clearance from your provider for postnatal exercise**

- **Arrange for childcare** (as applicable)

- **Create a will** – if you have a lawyer, great; otherwise, you could also look into online services (e.g., Willing.com, or check with your employer to see if you have access to any group purchasing discounts related to estate planning)

- Consider getting **life insurance** – check with your employer to see if you're covered under a group term life insurance policy as part of your employee benefits

- Consider various **financial and college savings strategies** (including starting a 529 plan, establishing a trust, opening a custodial individual retirement account (IRA) or Roth IRA)

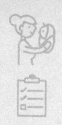

Chapter 43

BABY BLUES

When I heard the stat that 70%+ of women have the baby blues after giving birth, I thought it wouldn't apply to me. But this is not about your disposition or genetics prior to being pregnant. This is about the hormones that are running through your body after delivery that cause you to want to burst into tears at the smallest thing. Within the first few weeks of postpartum, I even joked with my partner about my "daily cry."

Baby blues can happen 2 to 3 days after you have your baby and can last up to 2 weeks. New moms may feel sad, moody, or cranky; cry a lot; have trouble sleeping, eating, or making decisions; and/or feel anxious and overwhelmed. These feelings are normal and usually go away on their own, but if they last longer than 2 weeks, or if you're feeling scared or out of control at any time, then call your provider immediately. Partners can help sense if something needs to be brought to the provider's attention. When in doubt, call and ask.

What may help you feel better?

- Know that as hard as today may seem, the challenges right now will not last forever.

- Really focus on self-care – they say to sleep when the baby sleeps. Try to do that as much as you can, and delegate (or ask your partner to help delegate) anything that doesn't absolutely require your involvement. Remember that the better state you're in, the better you'll be able to take care of your newborn. Babies can sense your stress. So, for your sake and theirs, prioritize your own physical, mental, and emotional well-being so that you can show up as best as you can for your baby.

- Social interaction helps, so either seek out a new mom's support group (your provider will have plenty of resources and ideas for you) and/or call your friends and family on video chat regularly.

- Take the pressure off yourself. Your baby's milestones are not a reflection of your parenting ability.

A NOTE ON POSTPARTUM DEPRESSION:

Postpartum depression isn't a character flaw or a weakness. And it's certainly not something to make light of or joke about. One in seven women will experience something more extreme than the typical baby blues. Postpartum depression can range from being mild to severe, and is treatable. Prompt attention and treatment can help you manage your symptoms and help you bond with your baby. If you have any questions, don't hesitate to call your health care provider and get the support you need as soon as possible.

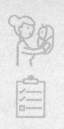

Chapter 44

INTERPRETING BABIES: BIRTH TO 3 MONTHS

In 2006, Oprah met Priscilla Dunstan, a woman who said she had unlocked what she called the secret language of babies. Her theory is that all newborns communicate by using five universal sounds, and that after listening to them a few times, mothers can learn to quickly identify each one and understand what their babies are saying.

"NEH" = hungry (sucking reflex)

"OWH" = sleepy (yawn reflex, oval-shaped mouth) (e.g., use pacifier)

"HEH" = discomfort (e.g., check hot/cold, uncomfortable position, change diaper)

"EAIR" = lower gas (more of an "ah" sound, tightened stomach, lower sound, often pulling legs up)

"EH" = burp (air bubble in top part of chest)

To see it in action, search YouTube for "One Woman Unlocks the Secret Language of Babies."

If you can't hear the difference, don't worry! There are only so many reasons a baby will cry. Check to see if any of these are relevant, and if still concerned, call your family physician or pediatrician.

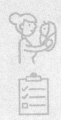

Chapter 45

EARLY
PARENTING DECISIONS

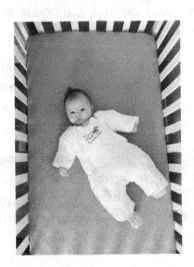

By now, you may have been given unsolicited advice from family, friends, or even strangers online about your baby. Just remember – what was best for someone else's baby may not be what's best for yours.

Your family physician or pediatrician is likely the best place to start for most questions . . .

"Is it normal for my baby to . . ."

- eat this much, sleep this long, or use this many diapers? (You may also want to consult a lactation consultant if breastfeeding.)

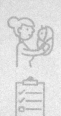

- cry this much?

- have this skin discoloration?

- have a tongue/lip tie? (You may also want to consult a pediatric dentist for a second opinion.)

"When will baby sleep through the night? What can I do to make that happen?"

- I know you'll hate hearing "it depends." But it really does – on your baby's own growth and development, on how your baby eats and spends his/her time while awake, on the physical environment, and more . . .

- When/if/how you choose to feed, impose a flexible schedule, sleep train, or anything else are parenting decisions that you'll have to make. A provider may inform your decision, but whatever you decide has to also make sense for your baby and your family unit.

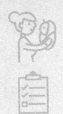

Chapter 46

BREAST OR BOTTLE?

The American Academy of Pediatrics (AAP) recommends that infants be fed breast milk exclusively for the first six months after birth, with continued breastfeeding until at least one year of age. Despite these recommendations, almost half of women in a 2018 Centers for Disease Control and Prevention (CDC) report had stopped breastfeeding at three months, even though the vast majority of them started out with the intention to breastfeed.

There are many reasons why new moms end up not following the AAP guidelines (e.g., sore nipples, inadequate milk supply – perhaps due to Cesarean birth, infant having difficulties, the perception that the infant is not satiated, difficulty pumping at work, other). It is not our place to judge others – but rather, to be informed about the pros and cons as we make a decision that is best for ourselves. Remember: It's your baby, your body, your business!

That said, if you've decided to give breastfeeding (and/or pumping) a go, then seeing an International Board Certified Lactation Consultant (IBCLC) you trust and getting a hospital-grade pump rental will give you the best chance of reaching your goals. (Even better, call your insurance company to find out who's in-network and if they'll cover the full cost!)

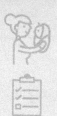

- Babies vary so much in their growth and development, and moms, too, vary a great deal in their ability to produce milk – that any Google search might just leave you even more overwhelmed and confused as to "what's considered normal." The truth is – what's normal is different for every mom and baby.

- Working with a lactation consultant will be well worth the cost, since you can expect to receive tailored guidance that helps you and your baby with your specific situation.

- You may have heard that milk doesn't just come flowing out immediately after you give birth. (You'll only produce very small amounts of colostrum in the first few days.) In order to allay your fears about inadequate supply to meet your child's needs, ask a certified professional how to build supply with the tools available to you.

SAMPLE QUESTIONS TO ASK A LACTATION CONSULTANT:

- How much milk is my baby taking when I feed?

- How much breast milk should I give my child if pumping and bottle-feeding?

- How often should I pump and/or feed, and how many times in a 24-hour period? Why? How should I expect this to change over time?

- When/what kind of pacifier can be used? Are there any you wouldn't recommend?

- What kind of bottle should I use to feed pumped breast milk? Are there any you wouldn't recommend?

- What is paced feeding? Why is it used? Would it be helpful in my situation?

- When might it be useful to take sunflower lecithin to help prevent clogged ducts?

- Any advice you have for moms who want to build supply before returning to work?

- Anything I need to know now about weaning?

- My goal is to: ___ (e.g., produce enough milk to feed my baby for the first year). What else do I need to know in order to achieve that?

HINT: The answer to many of these questions will depend on your goals, your body, and your baby – another reason why going by what you hear others do or what you find online is <u>not</u> advised.

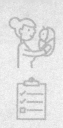

Chapter 47

SAMPLE BABY ANNOUNCEMENT

I almost didn't include this topic at all in this book. At first, I thought, "How does announcing baby's arrival have anything to do with the mom's health?!" Surprisingly, the drama of baby announcements gone wrong came up more than just a few times during the course of my interviews.

Today's social media norms vary by platform, generation, and culture. Sleep-deprived moms who have just undergone labor and delivery are in no state to think rationally about sharing the news about baby, much less consider the unspoken expectations that family and friends may or may not have related to who hears the news first and how. It's less important how you announce the arrival of your precious little one, and more important that you've given some thought to this topic in advance, perhaps even setting your expectations with family and close friends to take the pressure off yourself post-delivery. The following is a sample of what has been helpful for others . . .

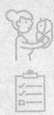

WHO TO INFORM, WHEN, AND HOW

- Within 1 Week: text photo to grandparents and siblings (and have them share with extended family)

- Within 1 Month: text photo to close friends (for example, wedding party) and email essential coworkers (e.g., your boss/team)

- Within 6 Months: send photo postcard to family and friends (e.g., wedding invite list) and/or share on social media

- Within 1 Year: 15 min video chats with different groups of family and friends to introduce baby

KEY INFO YOUR LOVED ONES MAY WANT TO KNOW

- Baby's full name
- Date and time
- Birth weight
- Size/length
- Birth location
- General health condition of mom and baby

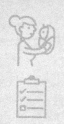

Chapter 48

CHILDCARE

For many people, the need for help with childcare is closely coupled with when their employers require them to return to work. There are often many factors we cannot fully control that impact our childcare decisions (e.g., length of parental leave, whether one or both parents can work remotely, who will be the primary caregiver during and after parental leave, proximity and availability of grandparents or other family members who can help, financial constraints, etc.) And, during a global pandemic, health and safety concerns become even greater obstacles to hurdle. Some may even weigh the question: "Should I leave the workforce for a period of time?"

For those who've decided that they would like help with childcare, and for whom friends and family aren't a sustainable option, it really boils down to two options: daycare or nanny. Being clear with what you want before you start the search will help you recognize the best option for you more quickly, which will serve you well in markets where demand for qualified help is greater than supply. Here are some additional questions to consider when making your list of pros and cons . . .

GENERAL CONSIDERATIONS

- What is the caregiver's general philosophy on childcare?
- Do they follow safe sleep practices?
- Will they honor your baby's sleeping and feeding routine?
- What kind of food do they serve?
- What activities will they do with your baby?
- How will they handle any unique requirements you may have? (e.g., strict diet, religious or cultural practices, special needs, medication needs, family/work situations, highly variable schedule, etc.)
- Do they have references you can contact?
- Do they offer a trial run?
- What's the minimum contract time period and/or cancellation policy?
- How do they measure success? How will you measure success? (e.g., safety, convenience, cost, etc.)
- What is your backup plan if your primary form of childcare falls through?
- Ideally when would you like to start? (Note that depending on where you live, there may be a 6–18+ month waiting list.)
- What does your intuition tell you?
- What can you afford?

DAYCARE

- Do I want the location to be closer to my office, home, or somewhere else?

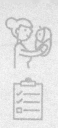
- Do they operate out of their home or other location? What security measures are taken at the facility? Is it clean and tidy?

- What are the child care licensing and regulations in your state, and do they meet/exceed those standards? (For more resources or to find child care in your state, go to: www.childcare.gov)

- Do you want them to have national accreditations for childhood development? (e.g., www.NAEYC.org, www.NAFCC.org)

- Does enrollment occur year-round or at certain times of year? Do they have a waiting list? When would they be available for your child to start?

- How do they select their caregivers? What training and vaccinations do their caregivers have? Will they take time to talk with you and answer your questions? What is the staff turnover rate? What is the caregiver-to-child ratio in the room your child would be in?

- What does a typical day look like for the room your child would be in?

- How often do you get updates about your child throughout the day?

- What happens if a nurse or medical care is needed?

- What's explicitly stated in their contract? (e.g., policies regarding days off and late pick up, visitors, sickness and immunization, etc.)

NANNY

- Do you want your own or do you want to share a nanny?

- Where do you want the nanny to take care of your child?

- Will your nanny live at your residence?

- What hours would you want your nanny to work?

- What's the time frame you'd like your nanny to be with your family?

- What other housework would you like the nanny to do? (e.g., baby laundry and sheets, dishes, food prep, light cleaning and tidying, pet and plant care, etc.)

- What training or vaccinations do you want your nanny to have? (e.g., high school degree, infant CPR and first aid, influenza, COVID-19, etc.)

- How will you find and select the nanny? (e.g., Care.com, agencies, personal referrals, vetting their experience via an interview and/or paid trial, conducting a background check, checking their driving record)

- Will you offer base pay, overtime, and paid time off for your nanny? What's the highest you'd be willing to pay in the event of a bidding war?

- How will you handle employment details? (e.g., taxes, paid time off, holidays; there are free nanny contract examples online as well as nanny payroll and tax services)

> Make sure you check to see if your employer offers the dependent care flexible spending account (DCFSA), which you can select during the annual open enrollment period to effectively lower your annual tax payment.

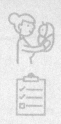

Chapter 49

SAMPLE SITTER INSTRUCTIONS

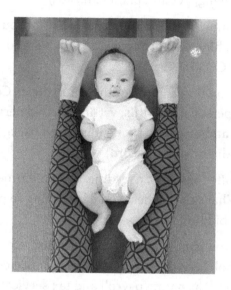

Not everyone has family and/or close friends who are able to help out, so consider yourself lucky if you do!

Whether it's hired help or not, here's a quick list of potential info you may want to share with babysitters, especially if it's been awhile since they've been around an infant.

1. **Contact info:** your and your partner's cell, your address, local hospital/pharmacy/police/fire/poison control center, family physician or pediatrician, trusted neighbor/ friends/relatives

2. **Medical info** about your child: allergies, health insurance, pediatrician's name and phone

3. Info about where the **first-aid kit** is located

4. **Inform the sitter**: put baby to sleep on back in bare crib, never leave baby unattended (especially on top of changing table or in the bathroom), never give baby honey (risk of botulism poisoning), never give any food or drink other than what is left specifically for baby

5. (If breastfeeding) **Breast milk instructions**: amount, how to pace the feeding when using a bottle, how to store and thaw breast milk (do not microwave milk or refreeze thawed milk) – for a printable summary, visit www.cdc.gov/breastfeeding/recommendations/handling_breastmilk.htm

6. Any info about the **baby's latest routine** (e.g., feed, play, nap, bath, bedtime, etc.)

7. **House rules** and any other **safety precautions** or expectations if going outside (e.g., sunscreen or hat, layers to bundle up in if cold, home before dark, childproofing – being especially careful about batteries that could pop out and other choking hazards, etc.)

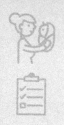

Chapter 50

BACK AT WORK HACKS

For those who decide to return to work at some point, here are some hacks many new parents have found to be helpful . . .

IDEAS AND TIME-SAVERS

- Cook bigger batches of food whenever preparing meals – there are lots of easy, inspiring, and nutritious sheet pan recipes online
- Order several take-out meals at a time (especially since there are now increasingly more delivery services and nutritionally-rich options available)
- Set up auto-ship services for essentials (e.g., diapers, toilet paper, pantry items, etc.)
- If breastfeeding, pump directly into storage bags (e.g., Kiinde), and refrigerate used parts in a Ziploc until you're able to wash them
- It can be super helpful to get into a routine of planning ahead for the week with your partner, including discussing when to block off time for individual self-care, Zoom calls with family and friends, date night, or even just Netflix and chill
- Speaking of date night, keep a jar of ideas you can draw from (with and without baby, depending on whether or not you have a sitter)

TACTICAL TIPS
(FOR THE OFFICE OR HOME OFFICE)

- Don't be too hard on yourself – give yourself time to adjust by easing back in (e.g., start your first day back midweek)

- Stock up on snacks and always have water on hand

- If breastfeeding, block off time on your calendar for feeding and/or pumping, and don't let anyone pressure you into rescheduling (Federal law requires employers to provide reasonable break time for an employee to express breast milk for her nursing child for one year after the child's birth each time such employee has need to express the milk.)

- If traveling, check out the Mamava pump and nursing finder mobile app to locate and unlock spaces while out and about, or, if needed, see if you can ship your pumped milk home using FedEx or Milk Stork

- Keep a large shirt or bathrobe on over your work clothes

- Block off time for eating lunch and taking short breaks throughout the day

- Communicate with your employer about what's critical versus what's nice to have, and set appropriate expectations with your colleagues

- Don't be afraid to ask your boss or other team members for their advice and support

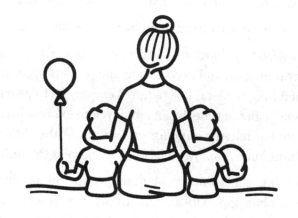

YAY! YOU MADE IT ALL
THE WAY THROUGH!

SHARE YOUR EXPERIENCE

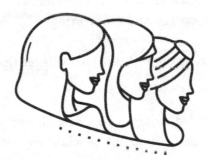

Did you find this helpful? I'd love to hear how this was for you!

What worked? How was your experience different?

Our collective experiences are powerful.

Let me know what additional wisdom you have that might make this unique time easier for other moms and moms-to-be.

Leave a review on Amazon to help others determine if this would be helpful for them or send me a note at:

www.joyandclaritylife.com

ACKNOWLEDGEMENTS

Thank you, Creator, for giving me the inspiration, strength, and willpower to finish this project.

To Mike, I love you and thank my lucky stars every day for your encouragement, energy, and unwavering support.

To Elly, for opening up my heart to be bigger than I ever imagined possible.

To my mom and dad, words cannot describe my gratitude for all you've done for me. I would not be who I am without your love and support.

To Lao Lao, Nai Nai, Da Gu Gu, Xiao Gu Gu, and my family in China for shedding light on what it means to "sit the moon."

To Carter Cast, Suzanne Muchin, Craig Wortmann, Haley Rolff, Nate Brown, The Garage at Northwestern, and Zell at Kellogg for being the first to believe in me and my startup ideas.

To the late Mr. Maier, my high school English teacher and coach, who would've been delighted to know that I had written a book.

To Cathy Suter, for her keen sense and eagle eye.

Many thanks to the late Donna Shenoha, industry thought leader and benefits strategist at Wells Fargo, for sharing her expertise and wisdom, even while undergoing cancer treatment.

I'm indebted to Daniel Martin, Brenda Booth-Ellington, Pete McNerney, David Schonthal, Greg Latterman, Ellen Havdala,

Rick Desai, Karin O'Connor, Rick Kolsky, Billy Banks, Mohan Sawhney, Harry Kraemer, Fred Matteson, George Jones, Jen Nelsen, Rashmi Kumar, and Dr. Tony Vancauwelaert for their mentorship and guidance. Many thanks to Melissa Kaufman, Neal Sales-Griffin, Moran Cerf, Linda Darragh, Sunny Russell, Elisa Mitchell, Sean Johnson, Bridgette Ferraro, Jennifer Herold, Elisa La Cava, Mia Velasquez, Dan Partida, Grant Wycliff, Josh Robinson, Adam Attas, Vivian Luu, Danielle Fox, Amanda Barber, Gamze Bilsen, Darren Green, Esther Barron, and Sandra Lopez for all of their help.

Thanks to Northwestern Medicine Prentice Women's Hospital, Northwestern Feinberg School of Medicine, Alberto Culver Health Learning Center at Northwestern Memorial Hospital, Swedish Hospital Nurse Midwifery Group, Midwifery and Women's Health at Elmhurst Clinic, 312 Doulas, DuPage Medical Group, North Shore Hospital, Sodexo Quality of Life Services, Yale New Haven Hospital, Jackson Memorial Hospital, UCLA Health, Hahnemann Hospital Philadelphia, T. Colin Campbell Center for Nutrition Studies at Cornell University, Cleveland Clinic, Columbia University Irving Medical Center, National Health Association, Department of Preventive Medicine at Northwestern University, Cedars-Sinai Medical Center, CHRISTUS Health, Hospital of the University of Pennsylvania, Penn Career Services, Career Management Center at Kellogg, Digital Health Division at the Israeli Ministry of Health, MATTER Chicago, and their staff for their gracious support and resources.

Thank you to the many independent obstetricians, midwives, doulas, nurses, pediatricians, perinatal mood disorder and women's mental health therapists, pelvic floor physical therapists, registered dietitians, lactation consultants, neonatologists,

neuroscientists, behavioral scientists, postpartum health practitioners and researchers, psychologists, therapists, social workers, executive and life coaches, and insurance, HR benefits, and
regulatory experts who shared with me their knowledge and
inspired me with their passion.

Finally, I'm eternally grateful to the many parents and support-
ers of the cause across the United States for their vulnerability
and willingness to spend time with me and share their stories,
wisdom, and expertise in the hopes that we may all realize a
future where all moms are as well taken care of as their babies.

INDEX

ABOUT THE AUTHOR

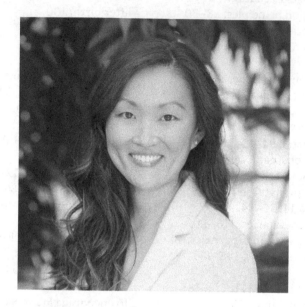

Dianna He Murray is a mom, executive coach, and healthcare industry veteran who helps leaders define and pursue what matters most. She is also a prenatal yoga instructor and certified in plant-based nutrition. In 2017, Dianna started a digital health company to improve maternal health outcomes, and saw first-hand the power of equipping women with the knowledge and tools they need to navigate the physical, mental, and emotional transition to motherhood.

Born in China, Dianna moved to the U.S. at the age of four, and has lived across the country, currently residing in the suburbs of Chicago with her husband and daughter. When she's not singing nursery rhymes with her baby girl, she loves to make delicious, nourishing food and be out in nature.